PROMOTING POSITIVE ADOLESCENT HEALTH BEHAVIORS AND OUTCOMES

Thriving in the 21st Century

Committee on Applying Lessons of Optimal Adolescent Health to Improve Behavioral Outcomes for Youth

Robert Graham and Nicole F. Kahn, *Editors*

Board on Children, Youth, and Families

Division of Behavioral and Social Sciences and Education
Health and Medicine Division

A Consensus Study Report of

The National Academies of
SCIENCES · ENGINEERING · MEDICINE

THE NATIONAL ACADEMIES PRESS
Washington, DC
www.nap.edu

THE NATIONAL ACADEMIES PRESS   500 Fifth Street, NW   Washington, DC 20001

This activity was supported by a contract between the National Academy of Sciences and the Office of the Assistant Secretary for Health of the United States Department of Health and Human Services (#10004318). Support for the work of the Board on Children, Youth and Families is provided primarily by grants from the Heising-Simons Foundation (award number is 2016-210), Jacobs Foundation (award number 2015-1168), and the Marguerite Casey Foundation (award number 2018-245). Any opinions, findings, conclusions, or recommendations expressed in this publication do not necessarily reflect the views of any organization or agency that provided support for the project.

International Standard Book Number-13: 978-0-309-49677-3
International Standard Book Number-10: 0-309-49677-2
Digital Object Identifier: https://doi.org/10.17226/25552
Library of Congress Control Number: 2020932720

Additional copies of this publication are available from the National Academies Press, 500 Fifth Street, NW, Keck 360, Washington, DC 20001; (800) 624-6242 or (202) 334-3313; http://www.nap.edu.

Suggested citation: National Academies of Sciences, Engineering, and Medicine. (2020). *Promoting Positive Adolescent Health Behaviors and Outcomes: Thriving in the 21st Century*. Washington, DC: The National Academies Press. https://doi.org/10.17226/25552.

The National Academies of
SCIENCES · ENGINEERING · MEDICINE

The **National Academy of Sciences** was established in 1863 by an Act of Congress, signed by President Lincoln, as a private, nongovernmental institution to advise the nation on issues related to science and technology. Members are elected by their peers for outstanding contributions to research. Dr. Marcia McNutt is president.

The **National Academy of Engineering** was established in 1964 under the charter of the National Academy of Sciences to bring the practices of engineering to advising the nation. Members are elected by their peers for extraordinary contributions to engineering. Dr. John L. Anderson is president.

The **National Academy of Medicine** (formerly the Institute of Medicine) was established in 1970 under the charter of the National Academy of Sciences to advise the nation on medical and health issues. Members are elected by their peers for distinguished contributions to medicine and health. Dr. Victor J. Dzau is president.

The three Academies work together as the **National Academies of Sciences, Engineering, and Medicine** to provide independent, objective analysis and advice to the nation and conduct other activities to solve complex problems and inform public policy decisions. The National Academies also encourage education and research, recognize outstanding contributions to knowledge, and increase public understanding in matters of science, engineering, and medicine.

Learn more about the National Academies of Sciences, Engineering, and Medicine at **www.nationalacademies.org**.

The National Academies of
SCIENCES · ENGINEERING · MEDICINE

Consensus Study Reports published by the National Academies of Sciences, Engineering, and Medicine document the evidence-based consensus on the study's statement of task by an authoring committee of experts. Reports typically include findings, conclusions, and recommendations based on information gathered by the committee and the committee's deliberations. Each report has been subjected to a rigorous and independent peer-review process and it represents the position of the National Academies on the statement of task.

Proceedings published by the National Academies of Sciences, Engineering, and Medicine chronicle the presentations and discussions at a workshop, symposium, or other event convened by the National Academies. The statements and opinions contained in proceedings are those of the participants and are not endorsed by other participants, the planning committee, or the National Academies.

For information about other products and activities of the National Academies, please visit www.nationalacademies.org/about/whatwedo.

Acknowledgments

We are grateful to many people for their support and contributions to this report. First and foremost, we would like to thank the study sponsor, the Office of the Assistant Secretary for Health (OASH) of the U.S. Department of Health and Human Services.

We would also like to thank the members of the study committee, who dedicated their time, energy, and expertise to the report. The committee also received significant contributions from several outside experts. Thank you to Robert Mahaffey (Rural School and Community Trust), Wesley Thomas (District of Columbia Public Schools), Sandra Shephard (Prince George's County Board of Education), Lisa Rue (cliexa), Ty Ridenour (RTI International), Elizabeth D'Amico (RAND Corporation), Aaron Hogue (Center on Addiction), Heather Hensman Kettrey (Clemson University), Kim Robinson (Forum for Youth Investment), Randall Juras (Abt Associates), Irene Ericksen (Institute for Research and Evaluation), and Jennifer Manlove (Child Trends) for sharing their work and expertise during our public information-gathering session. We also would like to thank the authors of our five commissioned papers: Cady Berkel (Arizona State University) for "The Role of Sexual Agency and Consent in Healthy Adolescent Development," Bethany Everett (University of Utah) for "Optimal Adolescent Health to Improve Behavioral Outcomes for LGBTQ Youth," Willi Horner-Johnson and Lindsay Sauvé (Oregon Health & Science University) for "Applying Lessons of Optimal Adolescent Health to Improve Behavioral Outcomes for Youth with Disabilities," Megan Moreno (University of Wisconsin–Madison) for "Adolescent Health and Media," and the University of Michigan MyVoice team for "Youth Perspectives on Being Healthy and Thriving." We are grateful as well to the following Teen Pregnancy Prevention (TPP) program Tier 1B grantees, who shared successes and challenges of program implementation in memorandums to the committee: the Baltimore City Health Department, the Mary Black Foundation, Methodist Le Bonheur Community Outreach, Morehouse School of Medicine, San Diego Youth Services, and the Center for Black Women's Wellness, Inc.

In addition, we would like to sincerely thank the youth who provided valuable input for this report. Thank you to Richard Nukpeta (Mentor Foundation USA), Shayna Shor (University of Maryland Health Center Peer Educator Program), and Natnael Abate (Promising Futures DC) for taking a healthy risk and sharing their experiences at our public information-gathering session. We also thank the MyVoice project participants, whose responses to our text message poll added important depth to this report.

This Consensus Study Report was reviewed in draft form by individuals chosen for their diverse perspectives and technical expertise. The purpose of this independent review is to provide candid and critical comments that will assist the National Academies of Sciences, Engineering, and Medicine in making each published report as sound as possible and to ensure that it meets the institutional standards for quality, objectivity, evidence, and responsiveness to the study charge. The review comments and draft manuscript remain confidential to protect the integrity of the deliberative process.

We thank the following individuals for their review of this report: Suzanne R. Bakken, School of Nursing, Columbia University; Claire D. Brindis, Philip R. Lee Institute for Health Policy Studies, University of California, San Francisco; Julianna Deardorff, Center of Excellence in Maternal, Child, and Adolescent Health, University of California, Berkeley; Phillip W. Graham, Center on Social Determinants, Risk Behaviors, and Prevention Science, RTI International; Norval J. Hickman, Tobacco-Related Disease Research Program, University of California Office of the President; Denese Shervington, Institute of Women and Ethnic Studies, New Orleans, Louisiana; Laurence Steinberg, Department of Psychology, Temple University; Benjamin W. Van Voorhees, Department of Pediatrics, University of Illinois at Chicago; and Janet A. Welsh, Bennett-Pierce Prevention Research Center, Pennsylvania State University.

Although the reviewers listed above provided many constructive comments and suggestions, they were not asked to endorse the conclusions or recommendations of this report nor did they see the final draft before its release. The review of this report was overseen by Rosemary Chalk, independent consultant, Bethesda, Maryland, and Bobbie A. Berkowitz, Columbia University School of Nursing (*emerita*). They were responsible for making certain that an independent examination of this report was carried out in accordance with the standards of the National Academies and that all review comments were carefully considered. Responsibility for the final content rests entirely with the authoring committee and the National Academies.

We are grateful to the staff of the National Academies, in particular to Richard Adrien and Rebekah Hutton, who provided critical research, writing, and editing support. To Pamella Atayi, thank you for the behind the scenes administrative and logistical support that was essential to our success. We would also like to thank Katrina Ferrara for her help during the editing process. In addition, we are exceedingly grateful to the Research Center at the National Academies, particularly Jorge Mendoza-Torres, for conducting our systematic literature search and fact checking this report.

Thank you to Natacha Blain, director of the Board on Children, Youth, and Families; Mary Ellen O'Connell, executive director of the Division of Behavioral and Social Sciences and Education (DBASSE); and Monica Feit, deputy executive director of DBASSE, who provided helpful oversight throughout this project. We are also grateful to Anthony Bryant and Faye Hillman for providing assistance in managing finances for this project. From the DBASSE Reports Office, we thank Kirsten Sampson Snyder and Yvonne Wise, who organized and moved this report through the review and production processes. In addition, we would like to thank Douglas Sprunger from the DBASSE Communications Office and Nicole Joy from the Health and Medicine Division Communications Office, who helped identify, plan, create, and execute our ideas for communication and dissemination. Finally, we thank Steve and Sarah Olson for their technical writing support and Rona Briere for her detailed editing.

Robert Graham, *Chair*
Nicole F. Kahn, *Study Director*
Committee on Applying Lessons of
Optimal Adolescent Health to Improve
Behavioral Outcomes for Youth

Contents

Summary

Adolescence is a critical developmental period in which youth grow, explore, learn, and develop important skills that prepare them for adulthood. While most youth navigate this period successfully, others may need additional support to be healthy and thrive. This support is often provided through prevention or intervention programs designed to promote healthy behaviors and outcomes from adolescence through adulthood. Accordingly, the Office of the Assistant Secretary for Health (OASH) in the U.S. Department of Health and Human Services requested that the National Academies of Sciences, Engineering, and Medicine convene an ad hoc committee to review key questions related to the effective implementation of the Teen Pregnancy Prevention (TPP) program using an optimal health lens. To carry out this review, the National Academies convened the nine-member Committee on Applying Lessons of Optimal Adolescent Health to Improve Behavioral Outcomes for Youth. In this report, the committee uses an optimal health framework to (1) identify core components of risk behavior prevention programs that can be used to improve a variety of adolescent health outcomes, and (2) develop evidence-based recommendations for research and the effective implementation of federal programming initiatives focused on adolescent health.

SELECTION OF BEHAVIORS AND RELATED OUTCOMES

This study's statement of task directed the committee to select the programs and outcomes to examine for inclusion in this report. Given the broad scope of youth risk behaviors and the limited time available for this consensus study, the committee chose to focus on three specific risk behaviors and their related health outcomes: sexual behavior, because the statement of task focuses on the TPP program; alcohol use, because, like sexual behavior, it is a behavior that becomes socially sanctioned with maturity; and tobacco use, because of the decades of research on prevention programs and interventions in this area that the committee considered to be informative to its task. However, the committee also noted important differences among these behaviors that limit comparisons of their respective prevention programs. In particular, while alcohol and tobacco are neurotoxic to the developing adolescent brain, sexual development represents a critical developmental task of adolescence that provides the building blocks for adult relationships. Thus, the committee recognized that, in contrast with the prevention of substance use, support for healthy sexual development is as important as prevention of the negative health outcomes associated with sexual behavior (e.g., unintended pregnancy, sexually transmitted infections) during adolescence.

THE OPTIMAL HEALTH FRAMEWORK

As a framework for this report, the committee used O'Donnell's definition of optimal health as "a dynamic balance of physical, emotional, social, spiritual, and intellectual health." Importantly, this framework stresses the influences of the physical and social environments, which for adolescents include parents, peers, schools, communities, and media. These factors, as well as the social determinants that drive them, either increase or reduce the likelihood of an adolescent's engaging in unhealthy risk behaviors. Given that the committee found only one definition of "optimal health" in the peer-reviewed literature, however, the use of this framework should not be interpreted as an endorsement of its use in adolescent health programming.

ADOLESCENT RISK-TAKING BEHAVIOR

Neurobiological changes that occur during adolescence influence young people to seek out novel experiences and make sense of their environments through exploration, experimentation, and risk taking, which help adolescents transition from dependence on parents or other caregivers toward independence and self-identity. Yet while risk-taking behaviors are a normal part of adolescence, adolescents are also more likely than members of other age groups to participate in unhealthy risk behaviors, such as unprotected sexual activity, binge drinking, and tobacco use. These behaviors can lead to outcomes that not only threaten an adolescent's own health but also can endanger others.

TRENDS IN SELECTED BEHAVIORS AND RELATED OUTCOMES

Demographic trends for these three risk behaviors are reviewed in the report using data from the Youth Risk Behavior Survey, a large, nationally representative sample of in-school adolescents that has been administered every 2 years since 1991. Health outcome data are drawn from the Centers for Disease Control and Prevention's surveillance systems, the U.S. Department of Transportation, and the National Survey of Family Growth.

Broadly, these data show that the prevalence of adolescent sexual behavior, alcohol use, and cigarette use has decreased over time, while e-cigarette use and vaping among adolescents have increased significantly in recent years. Importantly, despite decreases in adolescent sexual behavior among all racial/ethnic groups, significant disparities remain in pregnancy, birth, and sexually transmitted infection rates—disparities that can be linked to differences in access to opportunities and supports. The committee therefore concluded that disadvantaged youth need more resources to reduce these disparities and ensure access to comparable opportunities.

CORE COMPONENTS OF PROGRAMS AND INTERVENTIONS

The committee was charged with identifying the key elements, or core components, that help make programs and interventions effective in improving outcomes for youth. Such components are defined as discrete, reliably identifiable techniques, strategies, or practices that are intended to influence the behavior or well-being of a service recipient. To carry out this task, the committee conducted a systematic review of systematic reviews and meta-analyses, focusing on programs aimed at promoting positive adolescent health behaviors and outcomes.

Few studies included in the committee's review were designed to identify and evaluate the effectiveness of specific core components. However, the committee's review did show the strengths of social-emotional learning and positive youth development programs that are provided from childhood throughout adolescence. These programs teach skills that, if learned successfully, underlie and impact a variety of health behaviors and outcomes across the life course by providing a foundation upon which other specific behavioral skills and services (e.g., understanding social norms around drugs, negotiating condom use, access to contraception) can be built. Furthermore, those programs that involve youth, families, and communities and that target social determinants of health have been shown to help reduce disparities in health outcomes related to social and economic disadvantage.

RECOMMENDATIONS AND PROMISING APPROACHES

Based on the results of the review described above, the committee arrived at three recommendations.

RECOMMENDATION 1: The U.S. Department of Health and Human Services should fund additional research aimed at identifying, measuring, and evaluating the effectiveness of specific core components of programs and interventions focused on promoting positive health behaviors and outcomes among adolescents.

RECOMMENDATION 2: The Division of Adolescent and School Health of the Centers for Disease Control and Prevention should

- update and expand the Youth Risk Behavior Survey (YRBS) to include
  — out-of-school youth (e.g., homeless, incarcerated, dropped out), and
  — survey items that reflect a more comprehensive set of sexual risk behaviors with specific definitions; and
- conduct further research on the ideal setting and mode for administering the YRBS with today's adolescents.

RECOMMENDATION 3: The Office of the Assistant Secretary for Health within the U.S. Department of Health and Human Services should fund universal, holistic, multicomponent programs that meet all of the following criteria:

- promote and improve the health and well-being of the whole person, laying the foundation for specific, developmentally appropriate behavioral skills development;
- begin in early childhood and are offered during critical developmental windows, from childhood throughout adolescence;
- consider adolescent decision making, exploration, and risk taking as normative;
- engage diverse communities, public policy makers, and societal leaders to improve modifiable social and environmental determinants of health and well-being that disadvantage and stress young people and their families; and
- are theory driven and evidence based.

The committee also identified two promising approaches that deserve more meaningful attention in the design, implementation, and evaluation of adolescent health programs.

Promising Approach 1: Programs can benefit from implementing and evaluating policies and practices that promote inclusiveness and equity so that all youth are able to thrive.

Promising Approach 2: Programs can benefit from including youth of diverse ages, racial/ethnic backgrounds, socioeconomic status, rurality/ urbanity, sexual orientations, sexes/genders, and disability/ability status in their decision-making processes.

1

Introduction

And for me, what I think a thriving person in 2019 is when you're physically, mentally, and emotionally stable. I feel like you accept yourself for who you are and you're around people that support you emotionally and you can in return give that support back.

Natnael Abate, age 18
Peer Educator with Promising Futures DC
Public Information-Gathering Session, April 17, 2019

Adolescence is period of immense growth, learning, exploration, and opportunity during which youth develop the knowledge, attitudes, and skills that will help them thrive throughout life. While most youth traverse adolescence without incident, some need additional support to promote their optimal health. Sometimes such support comes in the form of a prevention or intervention program designed to capitalize on the rapid, formative changes that occur during this period so as to encourage healthy behaviors that will follow the adolescent through adulthood. However, no program is one size fits all, and too often these programs target specific risk behaviors instead of aiming to support the whole person. Such programs fail to understand not only the interdependence of health behaviors and outcomes but also the diverse needs and experiences of youth. In the face of the constant technological and cultural changes that define each generation of adolescents, moreover, the design, implementation, and evaluation of adolescent health programming will need to be more innovative to ensure the equitable achievement of optimal health for all youth.

STUDY OVERVIEW

In this context, the Office of the Assistant Secretary for Health (OASH) in the U.S. Department of Health and Human Services (HHS) requested that the National Academies of Sciences, Engineering, and Medicine convene an ad hoc committee to review key questions related to the implementation of the Teen Pregnancy Prevention (TPP) program using an optimal health lens. To carry out this review, the National Academies convened the nine-member Committee on Applying Lessons of Optimal Adolescent Health to Improve Behavioral Outcomes for Youth; the committee's full statement of task is presented in Box 1-1. The committee's membership, based on the study's statement of task, included expert scholars and practitioners representing a diverse set of disciplines, including program implementation and evaluation, public health, adolescent health policy and research,

---

BOX 1-1
Statement of Task

The National Academies of Sciences, Engineering, and Medicine will convene an ad hoc committee to review key questions related to the effective implementation of the Teen Pregnancy Prevention (TPP) program. The committee, using an optimal health lens, will explore the scientific and public health literature surrounding key elements or core components effective in improving behavioral outcomes for youth. Specifically, the committee will analyze components of a variety of youth programs which may be successful in preventing adolescent-risk behaviors with the parallel goal of accelerating progress toward the discontinuation (and not merely the reduction) of those risks among currently engaged adolescents. The committee will identify the programs and outcomes to review and examine which factors contribute to optimal health. In addition, the committee will consider broader issues of methodology as they relate to examining specific components of programs in comparison to research that uses the program as the unit of analysis.

The report will recommend a research agenda that incorporates a focus on optimal health for youth. The report will also offer recommendations on ways that the Office of the Assistant Secretary for Health (OASH) can use its role to foster the adoption of promising elements of youth-focused programs in the initiatives it oversees such as mental and physical health, adolescent development, and reproductive health and teen pregnancy. Drawing on lessons learned, the report will present recommendations on ways OASH youth-focused programs could be improved.

psychology, public policy, teen pregnancy prevention, and health disparities. In this report, the committee uses an optimal health framework to (1) identify core components of risk behavior prevention programs that can be used to improve a variety of adolescent health outcomes, and (2) develop evidence-based recommendations for research and the effective implementation of federal programming initiatives focused on adolescent health.

The committee's statement of task reflects the sponsor's mission to integrate the concept of optimal health into its projects and initiatives, particularly those related to sexual and reproductive health (HHS, 2019a). OASH's "optimal health model," also referred to as risk avoidance theory (HHS, 2018a), indicates that optimal health is achieved when one is in a state of "no risk" (HHS, 2019a). Citing the public health prevention framework (described in the section on definitions later in this chapter), this model posits that optimal health can be achieved through primary prevention, or risk avoidance, and secondary prevention, or risk reduction, with the goal of always moving toward an area of lower or no risk. As originally applied to sexual behavior, risk avoidance refers to refraining from non-marital sexual activity (HHS, 2017a, 2018a), while risk reduction entails choosing to return to a state of risk avoidance or, if continuing to engage in sexual activity, using protection and family planning methods (HHS, 2019a).

In addition to adopting an optimal health lens for this project, OASH asked the committee to identify what could be learned from other risk behavior programs that could be applied to the initiatives it oversees, including not only the TPP program, but also programs focused on mental and physical health, adolescent development, and reproductive health more broadly. To this end, the committee was charged with using a core components approach, a relatively new program evaluation methodology that is already being used in other federal research and evaluation initiatives (Blase and Fixsen, 2013). Briefly, the purpose of core components research is to identify the "active ingredients" of evidence-based programs (EBPs) or interventions instead of evaluating a program as a whole. Once identified, these effective components can be used to implement programs more flexible than the original EBPs, which are often difficult to replicate with fidelity and inflexible to diverse community needs (Blase and Fixsen, 2013). With regards to the present study, the identification of core components that are effective across health behaviors and programs may also help in coordinating programming efforts in areas in which funding has historically been fragmented (e.g., teen pregnancy, substance use) (HHS, 2018b).

BRIEF OVERVIEW OF THE
TEEN PREGNANCY PREVENTION PROGRAM

The TPP program is a national grant program established by congressional mandate in 2010 under the direction of OASH's Office of Adolescent Health (now Office of Population Affairs). The purpose of this program is to fund organizations to develop and implement medically accurate and age-appropriate EBPs focused on preventing teen pregnancy among 10- to 19-year-old adolescents. Grantees are given 5 years of funding, and grantmaking is directed toward populations that experience the greatest disparities in teen pregnancy and birth rates.

The first cohort (fiscal 2010 to 2014) included 102 grantees, which collectively worked with approximately 500,000 youth across the United States. The second cohort (fiscal 2015 to 2019) included 84 grantees. Each grant fell under one of four categories focused on preventing teen pregnancy, the majority of which focused on replicating the effects of EBPs that were included in the TPP registry of effective programs. The four categories were (1) capacity building for EBPs (Tier 1A), (2) implementing EBPs to scale (Tier 1B), (3) early innovation (Tier 2A), and (4) rigorous evaluation of new approaches (Tier 2B) (HHS, 2017b).

STUDY APPROACH

An important part of the committee's charge was to explore the scientific literature on adolescent health behavior programs through an optimal health lens. Thus, the committee first needed to apply the definition of optimal health to the adolescent population and explain adolescent development through this lens. To this end, the committee drew on the National Academies report titled *The Promise of Adolescence: Realizing Opportunity for All Youth* (National Academies of Sciences, Engineering, and Medicine [NASEM], 2019a), as well as other evidence from established theories of adolescent health and development in the scientific literature (Chapter 2).

This study's statement of task also directed the committee to select the programs and outcomes to examine for inclusion in this report. Given the broad scope of outcomes that could be considered, the focus on risk behavior in the statement of task, and the limited time period for the preparation of this report, we chose to focus on three specific risk behaviors and their related health outcomes: ultimately, we selected alcohol use, tobacco use, and sexual behavior.

In general, these selections were based on (1) the prevalence of these behaviors among today's adolescents, (2) the significant amount of data describing demographic trends in these behaviors, and (3) the large number of peer-reviewed studies of EBPs that have targeted these behaviors and related outcomes. These three areas are not meant to provide exhaustive coverage of all the behaviors and health outcomes that are critical to optimal adolescent health. Rather, they are representative of the challenges that adolescents face and are well suited to review in a consensus study review because of their extensive coverage in the literature. More specifically, we chose sexual behavior given the focus in the statement of task on the TPP program. We selected alcohol use because, like sexual behavior, it is a risk behavior that is age graded; that is, it is generally considered to be socially acceptable once a person reaches a particular age or developmental milestone, rather than consistently considered to be a dangerous or unhealthy behavior across the lifespan. Finally, we chose tobacco use based on the decades of research on primary and secondary prevention programs for nicotine addiction and tobacco-related diseases, which we judged to be potentially informative to our task.

This approach is not without limitations. For example, we did not include a specific focus on obesity prevention programs relevant to healthy diet and physical activity, as the focus of our task was explicitly on risk behaviors. In addition, we did not include a focused review of programs to prevent violence. We made this decision in recognition of the wide breadth of topics that fall under the umbrella of violence, so that we were concerned that the scope of this literature would make it difficult to review and incorporate concisely in this report.[1] However, it is important to note that violence often co-occurs with our three selected risk behaviors. For example, violence in the form of bullying can lead to increased substance use behaviors, and sexual behavior under the influence of alcohol can lead to violence in the form of sexual assault. Thus where relevant, we draw connections to violence in our discussion of alcohol use, tobacco use, and sexual behavior.

Importantly, although many comparisons can be drawn among prevention and intervention programs for sexual behavior, alcohol use, and tobacco use, there are also significant differences that need to be addressed. For example, while we chose to focus on alcohol use because it becomes socially sanctioned with maturity, this does not mean that alcohol use and sexual behavior should be interpreted as analogous. Alcohol misuse represents a significant public health problem in the United States (Centers for Disease Control and Prevention [CDC], 2019a), and like tobacco, alcohol is neurotoxic to the developing adolescent brain (Institute of Medicine, 2015; National Research Council and Institute of Medicine, 2004). In contrast, sexual development represents a critical developmental task of adolescence, whereby the necessary building blocks for adult relationships are estab-

---

[1]See Box 3-1 in Chapter 3 for a list of recent National Academies reports dedicated to violence-related topics.

lished (NASEM, 2019a). It is therefore as important to support healthy sexual development as to prevent the negative health outcomes associated with sexual behavior (e.g., unintended pregnancy, sexually transmitted infections) during the adolescent period.

Chapters 2 and 3 of the report provide the groundwork for the committee's response to its central charge: to use evidence from a variety of youth-serving programs to identify key program factors that can promote optimal adolescent health. These chapters are based on the committee's examination of the scientific literature on adolescent development and risk-taking behaviors. To the extent possible, we cite recent reviews of the scientific literature rather than individual studies in these chapters in an effort to present information that is supported by evidence from multiple rigorous scientific studies and across contexts.

In developing Chapter 4, the committee used a systematic review methodology and expert review of contemporary papers on core program components to analyze the available research on adolescent health behavior programs using an optimal health lens. This review was intended to identify the core components of programs with evidence of effectiveness, with consideration of methodological issues. We also considered other methods for our review of effective program components, including a meta-analysis of primary studies, but eventually selected our systematic review approach as a way of examining a larger body of literature within the constraints of the study period.

Broadly, programs were included in our systematic review if they targeted outcomes in one or more of the five optimal health domains (physical, emotional, social, spiritual, and intellectual), with a particular emphasis on programs focused on alcohol use, tobacco use, and sexual behavior in the physical health domain. In addition to this systematic review, we reviewed contemporary papers that are clearly focused on core components of effective programs to ensure that we would examine the most current research on core components of adolescent health behavior programs.

Finally, the committee was asked to develop evidence-based recommendations for (1) adolescent health research and (2) the effective implementation of federal programming initiatives. Our resulting three recommendations and two promising approaches (Chapter 5) are based on the findings and conclusions presented in Chapters 2–4. While these recommendations and approaches are directed largely to federal, state, and local governments, and specifically to OASH offices and program grantees, other audiences of interest include professional associations for adolescent care, program providers, researchers, and community-based stakeholders.

To supplement our members' own expertise, we commissioned several papers; held a public information-gathering session; and requested information from current TPP Tier 1B grantees in order to hear from researchers, practitioners, educators, and youth on key topics related to our charge. We also commissioned a text message poll administered to a national sample of adolescents through the University of Michigan's MyVoice study. Major themes and selected quotes from this poll appear throughout this report to provide a youth perspective on what it means to thrive today. The full MyVoice report can be found in our online resources;[2] the MyVoice methodology is described in Appendix B.

DATA SOURCES

This section briefly describes the sources of data used by the committee and the rationale for their selection for use in this report.

The health outcome data derive from a variety of federal sources, including the CDC's surveillance systems, the U.S. Department of Transportation, and the National Survey of Family Growth (NSFG). To evaluate risk behavior trends, the committee deliberated over a number of nationally representative datasets—Monitoring the Future (MTF), the National Youth Tobacco Survey (NYTS), the National Survey on Drug Use and Health (NSDUH), the NSFG, and the Youth Risk Behavior Survey (YRBS)—that could provide information about adolescent alcohol use, tobacco use, and sexual behavior.

The MTF, NYTS, and NSDUH surveys all focus on substance use behaviors. More specifically, the MTF is a school-based survey funded by the National Institute on Drug Abuse that has collected data on adolescent drug use and related behaviors in every year since 1991 (Institute for Social Research, 2019). Similarly, the NYTS is a school-based survey that has been administered by the CDC every 1–3 years since 1999 to examine youth tobacco use and associated predictors and attitudes (CDC, 2019b; HHS, 2019b). Finally, the NSDUH is an annual household survey that has been administered by the Substance Abuse and Mental Health Services Administration since 1971, in which all household members ages 12 and older provide information about their alcohol, tobacco, and illicit drug use (HHS, 2019c).

In contrast, the CDC's NSFG is a continuous, household-based survey that has collected detailed data on family life, marriage and divorce, pregnancy, infertility, use of contraception, and general and reproductive health among those ages 15–49 since 1973 (CDC, 2019c). From 1973 to 2002,

---

[2]See MyVoice (2019). Youth perspectives on being healthy and thriving. *Report Commissioned by the Committee on Applying Lessons of Optimal Adolescent Health to Improve Behavioral Outcomes for Youth.* Available: https://www.nap.edu/resource/25552/Youth%20 Perspectives%20on%20Being%20Healthy%20and%20Thriving.pdf.

the NSFG included only women ages 15–44, but it has since expanded to include men (in 2002) and those ages 45–49 (in 2015).

The purpose of the Youth Risk Behavior Surveillance System (YRBSS) is to monitor the prevalence of a variety of health behaviors among U.S. adolescents that are associated with later morbidity and mortality outcomes, including behaviors that contribute to unintentional injuries and violence; sexual behaviors related to unintended pregnancy and sexually transmitted diseases; alcohol, tobacco, and other drug use; unhealthy dietary behaviors; and inadequate physical activity (CDC, 2018). Every 2 years since 1991, it has collected data from a nationally representative, cross-sectional sample of in-school adolescents who were in grades 9–12 during the study year using the national YRBS. More than 4.4 million adolescents have participated in the YRBS since 1991, with the most recent survey being conducted in 2017.

In reality, none of the currently available national datasets provide a fully comprehensive picture of youth risk behaviors, as all but the NSDUH and NSFG are school-based surveys. Thus they fail to include adolescents who are incarcerated; homeless; home-schooled; or in private alternative, special education, or vocational schools. This is a critical limitation, since out-of-school adolescents, particularly incarcerated and homeless youth, are at the greatest risk for engaging in unhealthy risk behaviors and are more likely to experience the related adverse health outcomes (Edidin et al., 2012; Odgers, Robins, and Russell, 2010; Tolou-Shams et al., 2019).

Among the above datasets, the YRBS is the only one that provides information on all three of the focal behaviors in this study (alcohol use, tobacco use, and sexual behavior) within the same group of adolescents. It is also the dataset that the sponsor identified as its main source of information about trends in adolescent risk behaviors. We therefore chose to use the YRBS to the extent possible to describe those trends for this report,[3] while also noting this dataset's strengths and weaknesses (see Chapter 3).

DEFINITIONS

The key terms used in this report are defined below.

Adolescence

Although the hallmark developmental changes of adolescence can begin before age 10 and persist after age 19, *adolescent* is defined in this report as

---

[3]E-cigarette data are from the NYTS because this survey provides the most up-to-date information on this rapidly growing epidemic.

a young person ages 10–19. This age range was provided to the committee by the sponsor and represents the target age range for the TPP program.

Optimal Health

The statement of task asked the committee to use an *optimal health* lens. After searching the current peer-reviewed literature for "optimal health" to provide this context, we found only reference to a definition by O'Donnell (1986). This definition was updated in 2009 as part of O'Donnell's broader model of health promotion, which he shared in an editorial statement for the *American Journal of Health Promotion* (2009) (see Box 1-2). This is also the definition that OASH has used for its optimal health model (HHS, 2018a, 2019a).

Since introducing the term in 1986, O'Donnell has written extensively about optimal health, providing detailed descriptions of each of its five dimensions (Box 1-2), as well as further interpretation of his original definition (2017). See Chapter 2 for further discussion of O'Donnell's optimal health definition.

BOX 1-2
Definition and Dimensions of Optimal Health

Definition
   "Optimal health is a dynamic balance of physical, emotional, social, spiritual, and intellectual health" (O'Donnell, 2009, p. iv).

Dimensions
   1. **Physical Health** is the condition of the body.
   2. **Emotional Health** is the ability to cope with or avoid stress and other emotional challenges.
   3. **Social Health** is the ability to form and maintain nurturing and productive relationships with family, friends, co-workers, neighbors, and others.
   4. **Spiritual Health** is having a sense of purpose, love, hope, peace, and charity. For some people, this is drawn from being part of an organized religious group; for others, it is having a sense of values inspired by other influences.
   5. **Intellectual Health** encompasses achievements in academics, career, hobbies, and cultural pursuits.

SOURCE: Excerpted from O'Donnell (2017, p. 76).

Adolescent Risk Taking and Experimentation

Neurobiological changes that occur during the course of adolescence influence adolescents to seek novel experiences and make sense of their environments through *risk taking and experimentation*. Although certain risk behaviors can have real and destructive impacts, adolescence is often wrongly viewed as being synonymous with a period of "storm and stress" (Arnett, 1999). Public perception of adolescent risk taking often entails negative connotations, such as the deep-rooted societal view that it is destructive. Instead, it serves as a precursor to the assumption of adult roles (Romer, Reyna, and Satterthwaite, 2017; Wahlstrom et al., 2010), helping adolescents become autonomous, explore their identity, and forge social ties (Maggs, Almeida, and Galambos, 1995). Risk taking therefore is a normal part of the transition away from a childhood state of parental or caregiver dependence to exploring and acquiring independence and self-identity (NASEM, 2019a).

At the same time, although risk-taking behaviors are a normative and adaptive part of adolescence, adolescents are more prone than those in other age groups to participate in *unhealthy risk behaviors*, such as tobacco use and binge drinking (Duell and Steinberg, 2019). Engaging in unhealthy risk behaviors can lead to adverse outcomes that not only threaten health, but also can endanger others, as in the case of reckless driving or violent aggression (World Health Organization, 2006). Accordingly, the impact of these unsafe behaviors on adolescent health outcomes has been recognized as an important public health issue (DiClemente, Hansen, and Ponton, 2013). Bearing the cost of these behaviors, society shares in the responsibility for helping to set adolescents on a path toward fully realizing their potential by promoting and improving their multidimensional health and by reducing the negative consequences associated with unhealthy risk behaviors through health promotion and prevention efforts.

Public Health Prevention Framework

The three-level *public health prevention framework* (Katz and Ali, 2009) was chosen as the initial model of prevention for this report based on discussion with the sponsor at the committee's first meeting. In this framework, *primary prevention* is focused on the risk factors for a disease or condition, with the intent of intervening before it occurs. Included in primary prevention are such interventions as vaccination and behavior change programs, both of which can prevent the onset or reduce the impact of a disease or condition (CDC, 2017; U.S. Preventive Services Task Force, 2018). *Secondary prevention* focuses on early identification of high-risk populations, which can aid in slowing or stopping the progression of a disease or condition (CDC, 2017; U.S. Preventive Services Task Force, 2018). It includes such strategies as early testing and monitoring for signs or symptoms of a disease or condition. Finally, *tertiary prevention* refers to treatment and rehabilitation after the onset or diagnosis of a disease or condition, which can prevent its future incidence (CDC, 2017; U.S. Preventive Services Task Force, 2018).

Importantly, this public health prevention framework is designed with *health outcomes* as the key target. Although a *health behavior* is an important predictor of a health outcome, behaviors are considered to be modifiable risk factors that are a focus in primary prevention activities and are distinguished from the health outcome itself.

This separation of health behaviors and outcomes is a subtle yet important part of this framework. Behaviors can be difficult to prevent, and societal attitudes and beliefs about the acceptability of such behaviors as alcohol use and sexual behavior often change with age. Thus, focusing only on avoiding or discontinuing these behaviors does not prepare a person to prevent adverse health outcomes once the behaviors are socially acceptable or age-appropriate.

For example, alcohol use during adolescence can have harmful effects on brain development, which has contributed to the adoption of laws regarding minimum legal drinking ages (HHS, 2017c). However, simply telling youth not to drink alcohol (health behavior) will not prepare them to avoid impairment and injury (health outcome) once this behavior is socially sanctioned. Instead, youth need to learn about the social norms related to drinking and how to make decisions about alcohol that can help prevent impairment or injury once their drinking behaviors are legal.

As another example, preventing an unintended pregnancy (health outcome) is an issue not unique to teens or unmarried people, as many people want or need to control their fertility after marriage. Therefore, an exclusive focus on teaching abstinence from sexual activity (health behavior) does not provide people with the necessary knowledge and skills to prevent an unintended pregnancy once they do have vaginal sex. Rather, targeting communication, decision-making skills, and family planning behaviors is more likely to be successful in preventing unintended pregnancy, not only during adolescence, but also across the life course.

Institute of Medicine (IOM) Intervention Classifications

As the committee began its review of programs and interventions (Chapter 4), we found that the *IOM intervention classifications* were another helpful way to conceptualize prevention for the purposes of our task. These classifications, based on the prevention model proposed by Gordon (1983), encompass universal, selective, and indicated programs and interventions.

Universal prevention programs and interventions target an entire population, regardless of its members' levels of risk. *Selective* programs and interventions target a subset of the population that may be considered at risk. Finally, *indicated* programs and interventions target those who are already beginning to experience the effects of a specific health outcome (IOM, 1994).

The public health prevention framework described above and the IOM intervention classifications are not mutually exclusive, but rather provide two different ways of describing prevention activities. Figure 1-1 illustrates how these two prevention models overlap. The half-moon in the center of the figure represents a health promotion model that was published in the most recent update (NASEM, 2019b) to the original IOM (1994) report. In this model, prevention is distinct from promotion, treatment, and maintenance. In contrast, the public health prevention framework, shown on the outer ring, takes a broader approach whereby promotion, treatment, and maintenance are included among prevention activities. The overlapping arrows in the public health prevention framework represent how program recipients may be at different levels of risk for the targeted health outcome when they receive intervention services.

Protective and Risk Factors

Programs and interventions that use these prevention models to decrease or eliminate negative health outcomes associated with unhealthy adolescent risk-taking behaviors often aim to capitalize on protective factors and mitigate risk factors (CDC, 2019d). *Protective factors* are characteristics of the adolescent or his or her environments (e.g., family, school, community) that help build resilience in the face of challenges. Research shows that adolescents who possess these protective factors are less likely than others to put themselves at risk for negative health outcomes by engaging in unhealthy risk behaviors (IOM, 2011). *Risk factors*, conversely, are characteristics of the adolescent and his or her environments that are associated with greater adversity and have been shown in research to be associated with more unhealthy risk behaviors.

Health Inequities, Structural Inequities, and the Social Determinants of Health

As described in a recent National Academies report (NASEM, 2017), *health inequities* are systematic differences in opportunities that lead to unfair and avoidable differences in health outcomes. There are two root causes of these inequities. First are *structural inequities* that result in an unequal distribution of power and resources based on race, gender, class, sexual orientation, gender expression, and/or other identities. These struc-

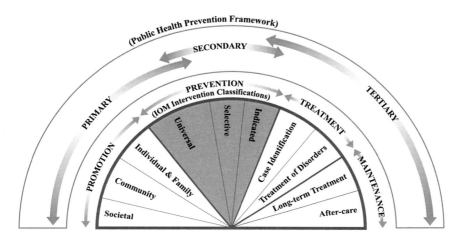

FIGURE 1-1 Overlap of two prevention models: The Institute of Medicine (IOM) intervention classifications and the public health prevention framework.
SOURCES: Institute of Medicine, 1994 (IOM Intervention Classifications); Katz and Ali, 2009 (Public Health Prevention Framework); adapted from NASEM (2019b).

tural inequities include, for example, such issues as racism, sexism, classism, ableism, xenophobia, and homophobia. The second root cause is unequal allocation of power and resources that results in unequal social, economic, and environmental conditions, which are also referred to as the *social determinants of health* (NASEM, 2017). The social determinants of health are defined as the environments and conditions in which a person lives, learns, works, plays, worships, and grows, all of which are influenced by historical and contemporary policies, laws and governments, investments, cultures, and norms (NASEM, 2017). While developmental changes help explain adolescent risk-taking behaviors, it is important to highlight the impact of these social determinants, as biological, behavioral, and social factors all play an important role in shaping adolescents' well-being, health outcomes, and exposure to risks (Acevedo-Garcia et al., 2014; NASEM, 2017).

To design and implement effective and sustainable interventions that reduce disparities and promote health equity, it is necessary first to understand how these social determinants affect adolescents—especially those who are disadvantaged and/or marginalized—and impede their health (NASEM, 2017). The effects of the social determinants of health are felt from the individual level (e.g., knowledge, attitudes, beliefs, and skills) to the systems level (e.g., policies, laws, and regulations) throughout the life course. These levels function both independently and concurrently, creating a complex social environment in which adolescents live and grow.

Studies have demonstrated the long-term protective effects of community socialization against such negative outcomes as deviant peer affiliation, conduct disorder, and unhealthy sexual risk behaviors (Browning et al., 2008; Nasim et al., 2011). Conversely, negative contexts can have deleterious effects on adolescents' well-being. For example, results from a meta-analysis of 214 studies on racial/ethnic discrimination and adolescent well-being revealed that elevated exposure to discrimination is associated with increased depression and other internalizing problems; greater psychological distress; poorer self-esteem; lower academic achievement and academic motivation; and greater engagement in externalizing behaviors, including substance use and unhealthy sexual risk behaviors (Benner et al., 2018).

Marginalization status is also an important consideration. For adolescents who are marginalized (e.g., those who are homeless, are justice involved, are estranged from their family, identify as LGBTQ, or have a disability), social, family, and individual exclusion can lead to health inequities. While marginalized groups are diverse, they share the likelihood of being people of color and lower-income, compounding the effects of structural inequities and negative social determinants of health that undermine their prospects for future well-being (NASEM, 2017). Marginalized adolescents have the capacity for resilience, but pathways for achieving health and well-being that target their needs must be available to them (Auerswald, Piatt, and Mirzazadeh, 2017; Institute of Medicine and National Research Council, 2015).

However, identifying these needs can be challenging. There is a major gap in the literature with respect to connecting behaviors that often lead to marginalization, such as juvenile justice involvement, compromised mental health, low school engagement, illicit drug use, early teen pregnancy, and sexually transmitted infections, to stressful conditions occurring in families. In addition, reaching and delivering services to many marginalized adolescents poses inherent challenges. Thus, those who are most in need of and might benefit most from interventions to reduce health inequities are often the least likely to receive them (Auerswald, Piatt, and Mirzazadeh, 2017).

Core Components Framework

Past federal programming has often required grantees to develop or use EBPs, programs that have demonstrated high levels of effectiveness based on (1) rigorous scientific evaluation, (2) large studies with diverse populations or multiple replications, and (3) significant and sustained effects (Flay et al., 2005). However, research indicates that EBPs are often difficult to implement with fidelity, which casts doubt on their effectiveness in diverse settings and populations (Barth and Liggett-Creel, 2014). As a result, more recent attention has been placed on the common, core components across a variety of EBPs, which may be more effective in improving targeted program outcomes compared with the program as a whole (Barth and Liggett-Creel, 2014; Chorpita, Delaiden, and Weisz, 2005; Embry and Biglan, 2008; Hogue et al., 2017). For this report, *core components* of programs and interventions are defined as "discrete, reliably identifiable techniques, strategies, or practices that are intended to influence the behavior or well-being of a service recipient" (Chapter 4).

ORGANIZATION OF THE REPORT

This report is organized into five chapters. Following this introduction, Chapter 2 focuses on normative adolescent development through an optimal health lens. Chapter 3 begins with a discussion of normative risk-taking behavior, then highlights demographic trends in alcohol use, tobacco use, and sexual behavior and their related health outcomes among adolescents. Chapter 4 presents the committee's review of the core components of adolescent health behavior programs and interventions, with a particular focus on the behaviors identified in Chapter 3. All of the above chapters end with a summary of the committee's chapter-specific conclusions. Finally, Chapter 5 presents the committee's three recommendations for research and programs/interventions, as well as two promising approaches for program and intervention improvement.

REFERENCES

Acevedo-Garcia, D., McArdle, N., Hardy, E.F., Crisan, U.I., Romano, B., Norris, D., Baek, M., and Reece, J. (2014). The child opportunity index: Improving collaboration between community development and public health. *Health Affairs, 33*(11), 1948–1957.

Arnett, J.J. (1999). Adolescent storm and stress, reconsidered. *American Psychologist, 54*(5), 317.

Auerswald, C.L., Piatt, A.A., and Mirzazadeh, A. (2017). *Research with Disadvantaged, Vulnerable and/or Marginalized Adolescents.* Florence, Italy: UNICEF Office of Research.

Barth, R.P. and Liggett-Creel, K. (2014). Common components of parenting programs for children birth to eight years of age involved with child welfare services. *Children and Youth Services Review, 40*, 6–12.

Benner, A.D., Wang, Y., Shen, Y., Boyle, A.E., Polk, R., and Cheng, Y-P. (2018). Racial/ethnic discrimination and well-being during adolescence: A meta-analytic review. *American Psychologist, 73*(7), 855.

Blase, K., and Fixsen, D. (2013). *Core Intervention Components: Identifying and Operationalizing What Makes Programs Work.* Washington, DC: U.S. Department of Health and Human Services, Office of Human Services Policy, Office of the Assistant Secretary for Planning and Evaluation.

Browning, C.R., Burrington, L.A., Leventhal, T., and Brooks-Gunn, J. (2008). Neighborhood structural inequality, collective efficacy, and sexual risk behavior among urban youth. *Journal of Health and Social Behavior, 49*(3), 269–285.

Centers for Disease Control and Prevention (CDC). (2017). *Picture of America: Prevention.* Atlanta, GA: Author.

———. (2018). *Youth Risk Behavior Surveillance System (YRBSS) Overview.* Available: https://www.cdc.gov/healthyyouth/data/yrbs/overview.htm.

———. (2019a). *Alcohol and Public Health.* Available: https://www.cdc.gov/alcohol/index.htm.

———. (2019b). National Youth Tobacco Survey (NYTS). *Smoking & Tobacco Use.* Atlanta, GA: Author.

———. (2019c). *About the National Survey of Family Growth (NSFG).* Available: https://www.cdc.gov/nchs/nsfg/about_nsfg.htm.

———. (2019d). *Protective Factors.* Available: https://www.cdc.gov/healthyyouth/protective/index.htm.

Chorpita, B.F., Delaiden, E.L., and Weisz, J.R. (2005). Identifying and selecting the common elements of evidence-based interventions: A distillation and matching model. *Mental Health Services Research, 7,* 5–20.

DiClemente, R.J., Hansen, W.B., and Ponton, L.E. (2013). *Handbook of Adolescent Health Risk Behavior.* Berlin, Germany: Springer Science+Business Media.

Duell, N., and Steinberg, L. (2019). Positive risk taking in adolescence. *Child Development Perspectives, 13*(1), 48–52.

Edidin, J.P., Ganim, Z., Hunter, S.J., and Karnik, N.S. (2012). The mental and physical health of homeless youth: A literature review. *Child Psychiatry & Human Development, 43*(3), 354–375.

Embry, D.D. and Biglan, A. (2008). Evidence-based kernels: Fundamental units of behavioral influence. *Clinical Child and Family Psychology Review, 11*(3), 75–113.

Flay, B.R., Biglan, A., Boruch, R.F., Castro, F.G., Gottfredson, D., Kellam, S., Mościcki, E.K., Schinke, S., Valentine, J.C., and Ji, P. (2005). Standards of evidence: Criteria for efficacy, effectiveness and dissemination. *Prevention Science, 6*(3), 151–175.

Gordon, R.S. (1983). An operational classification of disease prevention. *Public Health Reports, 98*(2), 107.

Hogue, A., Bobek, M., Dauber, S., Henderson, C.E., McLeod, B.D., and Southam-Gerow, M.A. (2017). Distilling the core elements of family therapy for adolescent substance use: Conceptual and empirical solutions. *Journal of Child & Adolescent Substance Abuse, 26*(6), 437–453.

Institute for Social Research. (2019). *Monitoring the Future: Drug Use and Lifestyles of American Youth (MTF).* Available: http://www.monitoringthefuture.org.

Institute of Medicine (IOM). (1994). *Reducing Risks for Mental Disorders: Frontiers for Preventive Intervention Research.* Washington, DC: The National Academies Press.

———. (2011). *The Science of Adolescent Risk-Taking: Workshop Report.* Washington, DC: The National Academies Press.

———. (2015). *Public Health Implications of Raising the Minimum Age of Legal Access to Tobacco Products.* Washington, DC: The National Academies Press.

Institute of Medicine and National Research Council. (2015). *Investing in the Health and Well-being of Young Adults.* Washington, DC: The National Academies Press.

Katz, D.L., and Ali, A. (2009). *Preventive Medicine, Integrative Medicine, and the Health of the Public.* Washington, DC: Institute of Medicine.

Maggs, J.L., Almeida, D.M., and Galambos, N.L. (1995). Risky business: The paradoxical meaning of problem behavior for young adolescents. *Journal of Early Adolescence, 15*(3), 344–362.

National Academies of Sciences, Engineering, and Medicine (NASEM). (2017). *Communities in Action: Pathways to Health Equity.* Washington, DC: The National Academies Press.

———. (2019a). *The Promise of Adolescence: Realizing Opportunity for All Youth.* Washington, DC: The National Academies Press.

———. (2019b). *Fostering Healthy Mental, Emotional, and Behavioral Development in Children and Youth: A National Agenda.* Washington, DC: The National Academies Press.

Nasim, A., Fernander, A., Townsend, T.G., Corona, R., and Belgrave, F.Z. (2011). Cultural protective factors for community risks and substance use among rural African American adolescents. *Journal of Ethnicity in Substance Abuse, 10*(4), 316–336.

National Research Council and Institute of Medicine. (2004). *Reducing Underage Drinking: A Collective Responsibility.* Washington, DC: The National Academies Press.

Odgers, C.L., Robins, S.J., and Russell, M.A. (2010). Morbidity and mortality risk among the "forgotten few": Why are girls in the justice system in such poor health? *Law and Human Behavior, 34*(6), 429–444.

O'Donnell, M.P. (1986). Definition of health promotion. *American Journal of Health Promotion, 1*(1), 4–5.

O'Donnell, M.P. (2009). Definition of health promotion 2.0: Embracing passion, enhancing motivation, recognizing dynamic balance, and creating opportunities. *American Journal of Health Promotion, 24*(1), iv.

O'Donnell, M.P. (2017). *Health Promotion in the Workplace* (5th ed.). Troy, MI: Art & Science of Health Promotion Institute.

Romer, D., Reyna, V.F., and Satterthwaite, T.D. (2017). Beyond stereotypes of adolescent risk taking: Placing the adolescent brain in developmental context. *Developmental Cognitive Neuroscience, 27*, 19–34.

Tolou-Shams, M., Harrison, A., Hirschtritt, M.E., Dauria, E., and Barr-Walker, J. (2019). Substance use and HIV among justice-involved youth: Intersecting risks. *Current HIV/ AIDS Reports, 16*(1), 37–47.

U.S. Department of Health and Human Services (HHS). (2017a). *Sexual Risk Avoidance Education Program (General Departmental-Funded) Fact Sheet.* Available: https://www.acf.hhs.gov/fysb/resource/srae-facts.

———. (2017b). *About TPP.* Available: https://www.hhs.gov/ash/oah/grant-programs/teen-pregnancy-prevention-program-tpp/about/index.html.

———. (2017c). *Underage Drinking Fact Sheet.* Bethesda, MD: Author.

———. (2018a). *Model on Risk Avoidance Theory and Research, Informing an Optimal Health Model, 2017 - Overview.* Available: https://www.acf.hhs.gov/opre/resource/model-on-risk-avoidance-theory-and-research-informing-an-optimal-health-model-2017-overview.

———. (2018b). *Adolescent Health: Think, Act, Grow® Playbook.* Washington, DC: Author.

———. (2019a). *Introducing the Optimal Health Model.* Washington, DC: Author.

———. (2019b). *National Youth Tobacco Survey.* Available: https://www.healthypeople.gov/2020/data-source/national-youth-tobacco-survey.

———. (2019c). *National Survey on Drug Use and Health (NSDUH).* Available: https://www.samhsa.gov/data/data-we-collect/nsduh-national-survey-drug-use-and-health.

U.S. Preventive Services Task Force. (2018). *Procedure Manual.* Available: https://www.uspreventiveservicestaskforce.org/Page/Name/procedure-manual.

Wahlstrom, D., Collins, P., White, T., and Luciana, M. (2010). Developmental changes in dopamine neurotransmission in adolescence: Behavioral implications and issues in assessment. *Brain and Cognition, 72*(1), 146–159.

World Health Organization. (2006). *World Health Organization Youth Violence and Alcohol Fact Sheet.* Geneva, Switzerland: Author.

2

Normative Adolescent Development

Living my best life would include being physically, mentally, and emotionally "fit" and striving every day to reach a sense of stability.

Male, age 17[1]

Adolescence is a dynamic period of growth and change. As described in the recent National Academies of Sciences, Engineering, and Medicine report *The Promise of Adolescence: Realizing Opportunity for All Youth*, adolescence is "a period of opportunity to discover new vistas, to form relationships with peers and adults, and to explore one's developing identity. It is also a period of resilience that can ameliorate childhood setbacks and set the stage for a thriving trajectory over the life course" (NASEM, 2019, p. 1).

This chapter begins by presenting the major conclusions of *The Promise of Adolescence*. It then reviews research in the five domains of optimal health—(1) physical health, (2) emotional health, (3) social health, (4) spiritual health, and (5) intellectual health—as they relate to adolescent development. While not an exhaustive review of adolescent development, this chapter highlights the influences that are most relevant to each domain of optimal health.

---

[1]Response to MyVoice survey question: "Describe what it would look like to live your best life." See the discussion of the MyVoice methodology in Appendix B for more detail.

CONCLUSIONS OF *THE PROMISE OF ADOLESCENCE: REALIZING OPPORTUNITY FOR ALL YOUTH* (2019)

Adolescence forms the critical bridge between childhood and adulthood, making it an ideal window of opportunity to promote positive development. As noted in Chapter 1, although adolescence is often considered a "dark and stormy" time, exploration and risk taking are in fact necessary parts of growing up. They allow adolescents to form their identities; become more autonomous; and develop new cognitive, social, and emotional skills required for success in adulthood.

During adolescence, moreover, connections within and between brain regions strengthen and become more efficient, while unused connections are pruned away. These changes in the brain thus provide opportunities for positive, life-shaping development and resilience in the face of past adversity. Conversely, this plasticity also makes youth more vulnerable to adverse experiences. In that sense, adolescence represents a unique and important opportunity to support youth and promote the behaviors and skills that are critical to growth and development. Yet despite the opportunity provided by the brain's plasticity during adolescence, for too many youth, the promise of adolescence is not being realized. Adolescents' access to opportunities and supports varies by age, race and ethnicity, socioeconomic status, rurality/urbanity, sexual orientation and gender identity, and disability status. Long-standing disparities have created an opportunity gap that leaves many adolescents in stressful, dangerous, disadvantaged, and isolated situations that can have lifelong effects.

Youth from disadvantaged circumstances therefore need more than equal access to resources; rather, to ensure access to comparable opportunities, these youth need *more* resources relative to their peers from more advantaged backgrounds. Determining what resources might be necessary requires understanding how best to support adolescents as they begin to navigate the challenges and opportunities of this period of development, enabling them not only to survive but to *thrive* during this period.

ADOLESCENT DEVELOPMENT ACCORDING TO THE FIVE DOMAINS OF THE OPTIMAL HEALTH FRAMEWORK

As discussed in Chapter 1, the committee found only one definition of "optimal health" in our literature search. This definition, first presented by O'Donnell in 1986 and later updated in an editorial statement for the *American Journal of Health Promotion*, describes optimal health as "a dynamic balance of physical, emotional, social, spiritual, and intellectual health" (O'Donnell, 2009, p. vi). The five dimensions are further defined as follows (O'Donnell, 2017, p. 76):

1. physical health: the condition of the body;
2. emotional health: the ability to cope with or avoid stress and other emotional challenges;
3. social health: the ability to form and maintain nurturing and productive relationships with family, friends, classmates, neighbors, and others;
4. spiritual health: having a sense of purpose, love, hope, peace, and charity; and
5. intellectual health: the necessary skills for academic achievements, career achievements, hobbies, and cultural pursuits.

An important strength of this definition is the understanding that health is not unidimensional, but comprises various dimensions of well-being that are constantly changing and interrelated. As stated by O'Donnell (2017, p. 76) in his later work, "It is not realistic to expect to reach that magic point of perfect balance and stay there. It is more realistic to seek opportunities for growth and think in terms of a process of striving for balance under changing circumstances." Importantly, this statement allows for change in the relative importance of each dimension given the time, place, and situation. In each of the five dimensions of optimal health, then, a person's health is constantly changing based on a variety of biological, social, and environmental factors. Though individual goals and motivations drive certain health behaviors, O'Donnell (2017) asserts that perhaps the greatest predictors of health behaviors are the physical and social environments in which people live. Hence, these avenues may provide the greatest opportunity for health promotion.

O'Donnell (2017) describes a number of reasons why the social environment is so influential. First, individual goals are influenced by socializing agents and places. Second, socialization governs the norms and pressures that people face. Third, socialization occurs primarily outside conscious thought, which often leads to a lack of awareness about how socialization influences values, priorities, and goals. Thus, the social environment is critically important because of its powerful influence on people's daily goals, choices, and behaviors.

Although O'Donnell did not intend his definition of optimal health to serve as a model for adolescent health, the concept of seeking opportunities for growth under changing circumstances has relevance for this developmental period. While adolescence is a period of growing autonomy and independence, the adolescent experience is also highly dependent on the individual, family, community, and societal context (see Box 2-1).

Of course, this definition is not without its limitations. First, not all of the five dimensions of optimal health are easy to measure. For example, anthropometric data or medical and psychiatric diagnoses can be used

BOX 2-1
Youth Voices:
Tell us about something or someone
that helps you live your best life.

In a recent MyVoice survey, adolescents were asked about something or someone that helps them live their best life (see Appendix B for more detail on the MyVoice methodology). The top 10 answers from the 913 responses received are shown in the figure below. Overall, youth most commonly cited support from family, friends, romantic partners, and extracurricular activities or hobbies.

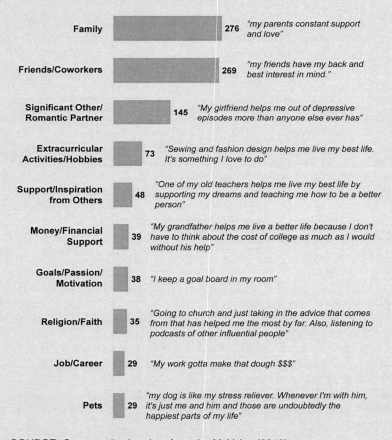

Category	Value	Quote
Family	276	*"my parents constant support and love"*
Friends/Coworkers	269	*"my friends have my back and best interest in mind."*
Significant Other/ Romantic Partner	145	*"My girlfriend helps me out of depressive episodes more than anyone else ever has"*
Extracurricular Activities/Hobbies	73	*"Sewing and fashion design helps me live my best life. It's something I love to do"*
Support/Inspiration from Others	48	*"One of my old teachers helps me live my best life by supporting my dreams and teaching me how to be a better person"*
Money/Financial Support	39	*"My grandfather helps me live a better life because I don't have to think about the cost of college as much as I would without his help"*
Goals/Passion/ Motivation	38	*"I keep a goal board in my room"*
Religion/Faith	35	*"Going to church and just taking in the advice that comes from that has helped me the most by far. Also, listening to podcasts of other influential people"*
Job/Career	29	*"My work gotta make that dough $$$"*
Pets	29	*"my dog is like my stress reliever. Whenever I'm with him, it's just me and him and those are undoubtedly the happiest parts of my life"*

SOURCE: Generated using data from the MyVoice (2019) report.

to measure various aspects of physical and emotional health, and school grades, educational attainment, and cognitive ability can serve as measures of intellectual health. In contrast, levels of social and spiritual health are much more difficult to measure.

Second, while the interactions among these dimensions make O'Donnell's definition attractive, they can make the dimensions difficult to tease apart. For instance, programs and interventions aimed at promoting adolescent health and well-being often focus on more than one dimension, as in the example of social-emotional learning. As a result, assigning such programs and interventions to one particular category can be virtually impossible. These measurement challenges are well illustrated in the review of programs in Chapter 4, where the committee was unable to identify groups of programs that fit exclusively into the social and spiritual health domains; instead, quite a few programs in the category of "multiple optimal health domains" include aspects of social and spiritual health.

Third, though adolescents typically reach a number of milestones in each of O'Donnell's five areas of optimal health, and while certain developmental progressions tend to occur during this period, adolescent development is also a highly individual process. This individuality creates some limitations in defining what constitutes normative development during this period. Defining stages and behaviors as "normative" can suggest that non-normative behaviors are negative; in the context of this report, therefore, the term "normative" is meant to align with typical developmental trajectories and milestones shared by youth of diverse backgrounds.

Finally, and in line with the aforementioned limitations, this report is, to our knowledge, the first to provide such a detailed examination of the literature on adolescent development and behavior using an optimal health lens. However, this review was constrained by the lack of definitions of "optimal health" in the peer-reviewed literature, and our use of O'Donnell's definition should not be interpreted as an endorsement of its application to adolescent health programming.

Each of the following sections is dedicated to one of the five optimal health dimensions. Each section first provides a description of important adolescent developmental milestones and trajectories for that particular dimension, followed by a discussion of the major social and environmental influences that affect those milestones and trajectories, including but not limited to parents, peers, schools, and media.

Physical Health

Developmental Milestones and Trajectories

In adolescence, puberty drives the primary physical changes that occur. These physiological developments, which include changes in a person's height, weight, body composition, sex characteristics, and circulatory and respiratory systems, are caused primarily by hormonal activity. Hormones prime the body to behave in a certain way once puberty begins and trigger certain behavioral and physical changes, and hormone production gradually increases until an adolescent reaches sexual maturation.

Although puberty typically follows a series of predictable physical changes, the onset and timing of these developments vary from person to person and have changed over time (Parent et al., 2016). Genetic, environmental, and health factors, including biological determinants, life stressors, socioeconomic status, nutrition and diet, amount of body fat, and presence of chronic illness, can all affect the onset and progression of puberty (Aylwin et al., 2019). Understanding the role of puberty is particularly important because pubertal hormones and the context in which they occur drive many of the motivations for novelty seeking that occur during adolescence.

Social and Environmental Influences on the Development of Physical Health

Bodily changes during puberty can have important effects on how adolescents perceive themselves and are perceived by others (NASEM, 2019). The physical changes that occur during puberty have been found to have as great an effect on an adolescent's self-image as the way he or she is treated and responded to by others (Graber, Nichols, and Brooks-Gunn, 2010).

Because adolescents experience puberty at different times and rates, their physical development can be a source of pride or shame. Parents and peers play a large role in shaping the attitudes of adolescents about their bodies and physical activity. Parents in particular can model healthy eating and physical activity and communicate positive messages about their child's appearance from an early age (Hart et al., 2015).

Schools have the potential to equalize access to opportunities for all students, as they provide an important environment for encouraging behaviors related to physical health, such as engaging in physical activity and eating a nutritious diet (Hills, Dengel, and Lubans, 2015). Schools can also provide a basic level of primary care services through school-based health centers (SBHCs). Indeed, research on SBHCs has demonstrated their effectiveness in delivering health promotion messages and services to young people, particularly those who may not have access to these services outside of school. SBHCs therefore represent an important venue for delivering health programming (Brown and Bolen, 2018; NASEM, 2019; Parasuraman and Shi, 2014). However, many schools struggle to implement high-quality programs that can drive positive physical health outcomes because of a lack of resources and institutional support.

Ultimately, many different genetic, social, and environmental factors affect physical development. The coordination of services and supports, as well as increased equitable access to resources, can help promote optimal physical health outcomes for adolescents.

Emotional Health

Developmental Milestones and Trajectories

Emotional health refers to the ability to cope with or avoid stress and other emotional challenges. In the past, adolescents have been characterized by their rapidly fluctuating emotions. Although researchers once attributed these emotions to the "storm and stress" expected in adolescence, these emotions generally reflect the interplay between the individual's social environments and the neurobiological and psychological changes that mark this period of development (Lerner and Steinberg, 2009).

In this report, the committee takes a strengths-based approach, viewing adolescence as an opportunity and indeed a critical time to help youth acquire positive skills related to emotion regulation. These skills interact with neurobiological and psychological changes to form the basis for the development of emotional health.

Neurobiological changes during adolescence Second only to infancy, the greatest neurobiological developments—many of which are associated with emotion regulation and decision making—occur during adolescence. Studies have found that the brain is extremely malleable during adolescence, with connections forming and reforming in response to a variety of experiences and stressors (Ismail, Fatemi, and Johnston, 2017; Selemon, 2013). This plasticity means that adolescent brains are highly adaptable to environmental demands. The onset of puberty spurs changes in the limbic system, causing greater sensitivity to rewards, threats, novelty, and peers; in contrast, the cortical regions, which are related to cognitive control and self-regulation, take longer to develop (NASEM, 2019). Theories of adolescent cognitive neuroscience suggest that this asynchronous development of these reward and control systems is responsible for adolescents' biased decision making and sensation seeking (Casey, 2015; Steinberg, 2014).

Psychological development during adolescence   In adolescence, youth must learn to identify, understand, and express emotions in healthy ways, also referred to as emotion regulation. A primary component of emotion regulation is the ability to handle emotions internally rather than externally. This includes recognizing how emotions impact thoughts and behaviors, learning to delay or reduce impulsive reactions to intense emotions, making decisions about situations based on how one might react emotionally, and engaging in cognitive reframing to change one's perspective on a particular situation (DeSteno, Gross, and Kubzansky, 2013).

Self-esteem (value judgments about oneself) is another critical aspect of psychological development and identity formation. Self-esteem is often at its lowest point in early adolescence, tending to improve in middle to late adolescence as teenagers become more emotionally mature. Differences between how one views oneself and how one believes one "should" be can lead to low self-esteem. Persistently low self-esteem is related to negative outcomes, including depression, delinquency, and other adjustment problems, in multiple optimal health domains (Allwood et al., 2012).

Adolescents are also at particularly high risk for developing many mental health conditions, including major depression, eating disorders, substance use disorders, and anxiety disorders (Herpertz-Dahlmann, Bühren, and Remschmidt, 2013; Merikangas et al., 2010). Beyond genetics, risk factors for these mental health conditions include exposure to, perceptions of, and reactions to stressors; elevated emotional and physiological reactivity; and developmental variation in the utilization of emotion regulation strategies (Carthy et al., 2010; Green et al., 2010; McLaughlin et al., 2011, 2012).

Social and Environmental Influences on the Development of Emotional Health

Pubertal hormones released during adolescence make youth particularly sensitive to stress (NASEM, 2019). These biological processes, combined with the heightened interpersonal stressors that occur during adolescence, are associated with disruptions in adolescents' ability to regulate their emotions effectively (McLaughlin, Garrad, and Somerville, 2015). Fortunately, an adolescent's social and environmental contexts can help mitigate the effects of stress. Adolescents who feel secure and protected in their immediate environments—home, community, and school—tend to handle stress more effectively than youth who feel unsupported, unsafe, or unprotected. Chronically stressful environments put youth at higher risk for depression, anxiety, alcohol or other drug use, teen pregnancy, and violence (NASEM, 2019). To handle stress and difficult situations effectively, adolescents must develop resilience—the capacity to recover quickly from difficulties. Resilience is developed through interactions within families, schools, neighborhoods, and the larger community (Zimmerman et al., 2013), which allow adolescents to practice dealing with stressful situations in safe and supportive environments. However, just as social support can help mitigate stress, adolescents who lack social support may be unable to develop confidence and effective stress management techniques (Compas, 2009).

Although disengagement from parents is common during adolescence, research has shown that parental relationships continue to influence important emotional outcomes (Branje, Laursen, and Collins, 2012). Research also has shown that family environments that support adolescents' expressions of autonomy are associated with a greater sense of agency and confidence in their own abilities, positive self-concept, and a sense of self-worth (McElhaney and Allen, 2012; Noller and Atkin, 2014). In cases where parents do not play central roles in adolescents' lives, natural mentors can serve as attachment figures and mitigate the risk for adverse outcomes (Dang et al., 2014; Thompson, Greeson, and Brunsink, 2016).

As illustrated earlier in Box 2-1, peers play a particularly important role in emotional development during adolescence. By middle to late adolescence, youth report relying more on either best friends or romantic partners than on parents for emotional support (Farley and Kim-Spoon, 2014). Although these interpersonal relationships can increase stressors and negative emotions, they can also, when of high quality, protect against the negative effects of such stressors and emotions (Farley and Kim-Spoon, 2014; Thompson and Leadbeater, 2013).

Schools also have the capacity to promote adolescent resilience by providing students with a sense of mutual responsibility and belonging (Epstein, 2011). Likewise, schools can help identify adolescents in need and provide services that can help. As with physical health, this role of schools is especially important for adolescents who may not have regular access to health care outside of school. In addition to such informal services as positive social interactions and emotional skill building, schools can provide formal services, such as counseling, that can improve both adolescents' social-emotional well-being and their academic performance (Brown and Bolen, 2018; Walker et al., 2010) (see Box 2-2).

Finally, social media have implications for adolescents' emotional health. Teenagers can use social media to express their emotions and opinions online, to seek social support, or to compare themselves with others. Research has found that adolescents who experience a greater number of positive reactions to their social media profile also experience higher self-esteem and satisfaction with their life (Ahn, 2011). On the other hand, misinterpreted communications, social rejection, and cyberbullying can have a range of negative emotional effects (Chou and Edge, 2012).

BOX 2-2
Youth Voices:
Specifically, what could your school do
to help you live your best life? (now or in the past)?

In a recent MyVoice survey, adolescents were asked about what their schools could do to help them live their best life (see Appendix B for more detail on the MyVoice methodology). The top 10 answers from the 886 respondents are shown in the figure below. Youth most commonly cited more school breaks, access to their passions, more real-world classes, improved social and mental health support, reduced costs, career and academic guidance, and a supportive school environment.

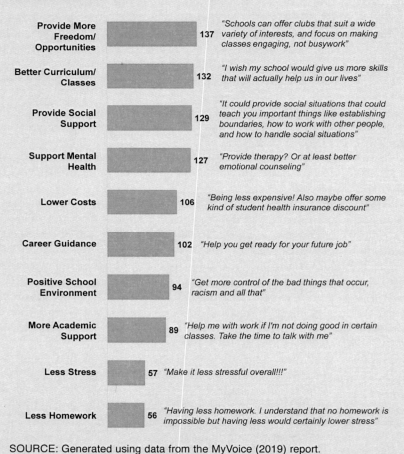

Provide More Freedom/ Opportunities	137	"Schools can offer clubs that suit a wide variety of interests, and focus on making classes engaging, not busywork"
Better Curriculum/ Classes	132	"I wish my school would give us more skills that will actually help us in our lives"
Provide Social Support	129	"It could provide social situations that could teach you important things like establishing boundaries, how to work with other people, and how to handle social situations"
Support Mental Health	127	"Provide therapy? Or at least better emotional counseling"
Lower Costs	106	"Being less expensive! Also maybe offer some kind of student health insurance discount"
Career Guidance	102	"Help you get ready for your future job"
Positive School Environment	94	"Get more control of the bad things that occur, racism and all that"
More Academic Support	89	"Help me with work if I'm not doing good in certain classes. Take the time to talk with me"
Less Stress	57	"Make it less stressful overall!!!"
Less Homework	56	"Having less homework. I understand that no homework is impossible but having less would certainly lower stress"

SOURCE: Generated using data from the MyVoice (2019) report.

Social Health

Developmental Milestones and Trajectories

Social health refers to the ability to form and maintain nurturing and productive relationships with others. As noted previously, adolescence is a period marked by increased autonomy. During normative adolescent development, most adolescents establish a level of independence and self-sufficiency that is marked by individuating from their family and beginning the important process of transferring dependencies from parental to peer relationships (McElhaney and Allen, 2012). An adolescent's social network can include friends, acquaintances, romantic partners, teams, and virtual communities. This social network continues to grow as adolescents seek out new experiences and engage in their community (Farley and Kim-Spoon, 2014).

Early adolescence tends to be marked by the most intense involvement in peer groups, with conformity and concerns about acceptance at their peak (Cowie, 2019). Although early adolescents experiment with romantic relationships, these experiences tend to be brief. Typically, early adolescents choose partners who align with the expectations of their social networks, reflecting their preoccupation with peers' perceptions of them (Cowie, 2019).

In middle adolescence, peer groups tend to become more gender-mixed. Adolescents begin to exhibit less conformity and greater acceptance of individual differences in this period, which is marked by a dramatic shift in multiple aspects of relationships, including number of relationships, length of relationships, and choices of partners (Bowker and Ramsay, 2018; Little and Welsh, 2018). They also begin what is more traditionally thought of as dating.

By late adolescence, one-on-one friendships and romantic relationships are often prioritized above relations with peer groups. Accordingly, the manifestation of romantic relationships between older adolescents reflects a greater interdependence between the partners than is the case in the romantic relationships of young adolescents (Bowker and Ramsay, 2018; Little and Welsh, 2018).

Social and Environmental Influences on the Development of Social Health

Compared with other age groups, adolescents are particularly influenced by the social norms of many groups, including family, friends, peers, virtual communities, and the broader society (McDonald, Fielding, and Louis, 2013).

The family is the first and primary social group to which most people belong, and parents represent important role models for the development of prosocial behavior (Hurd, Wittrup, and Zimmerman, 2018). As adolescents continue to develop more agency, this socialization process moves from being unidirectional (i.e., parent to child) to a more bidirectional, mutually beneficial process, characterized by discussion and negotiation of attitudes, beliefs, and practices (Smetana, Robinson, and Rote, 2015).

As discussed earlier, peer norms become particularly influential during adolescence. Positive peer modeling and awareness of peer norms have been found to be protective against violence, substance misuse, and unhealthy sexual risk (Viner et al., 2012). In contrast, social isolation, peer rejection, and bullying are associated with numerous unhealthy risk behaviors and adverse health outcomes, such as increased delinquency, depression, numbers of suicide attempts, and low self-esteem (Smokowski and Evans, 2019).

Schools also play a prominent role in the development of social health. In school, youth learn to relate with peers and form relationships with adult role models. For adolescents, a strong sense of attachment, bonding, and belonging; a feeling of being cared about; and a perception of teacher fairness are key factors in developing positive relationships with their teachers and their schools. Adolescents also tend to feel more motivated and engaged in school when they have strong, supportive relationships with their peers and teachers (Bakadorova and Raufelder, 2017; Wang and Eccles, 2013).

Perhaps the greatest social environmental influence on today's adolescents is social media. Social media add another layer to adolescent identity development, as adolescents must shape their virtual identities by determining what information to disclose online and where to disclose it (Boz, Uhls, and Greenfield, 2016). Social media platforms have also changed the ways in which adolescents relate to one another, increased the amount of time youth stay connected to one another, and redefined the meaning of friendship. Research has found that youth use such technologies as social media platforms to mediate their relationships with friends, romantic partners, and broader groups of peers (Nesi, Choukas-Bradley, and Prinstein, 2018) (see Box 2-3).

Although there are correlations between sociodemographics and particular social media communities, overall social media use is consistent across levels of household income and parents' educational attainment. Overall, 88 percent of teens report having access to a desktop or laptop computer at home, ranging from 75 percent among those from households with an annual income of $30,000 or less to 96 percent among those from households with an annual income of $75,000 or more. Moreover, as mentioned in Box 2-3, 95 percent of all teens report having access to a smartphone, a figure that has increased by 22 percent since 2014–2015. Interestingly, there is even less variation in smartphone relative to computer access by

---

BOX 2-3
Generation Z and the Role of Media

Adolescents identified as "Generation Z" (Gen Z—those born in the mid-1990s to mid-2000s) (Dimock, 2019) are the first truly "digital generation" that grew up surrounded by communication technologies and are accustomed to being both consumers and creators of media (Madden, 2017). This current cohort of adolescents therefore has unique experiences that affect their current and future health behaviors and outcomes.

Gen Z adolescents were children during the global rise of the Web, the Internet, smartphones, laptops, freely available networks, and digital media. Because they were raised with these technologies, they were able to internalize the newly connected world instead of having to adopt and adapt to it as did older generations (Seemiller and Grace, 2018). Today, use of social media is nearly ubiquitous among U.S. adolescents. Recent reports indicate that 95 percent of 13- to 17-year-olds in the United States have a smartphone or access to one, and 71 percent use at least one social media platform (Anderson and Jiang, 2018; Barry et al., 2017).

The bulk of research on the role of social media in adolescent health to date has focused on displays of risky content and the potential influence of this online content on adolescent behavior offline. Only very recently has there been a shift toward seeking a better understanding of how social media may promote wellness, healthy behaviors, or optimal health (Wong, Merchant, and Moreno, 2014). Further work is needed in this area, including studies that fully harness the social aspects of social media by studying interactions among peers, the distribution of content through a social network, or content posted on different platforms. There are also opportunities to engage youth in this process so as to understand their perceptions and interpretations, and to involve them in generating solutions (Liang, Commins, and Duffy, 2010; Moreno et al., 2018). Such studies would provide a better understanding of how health-related content is distributed and shared through social networks, and potentially help identify ways of linking social media and offline approaches to implement successful interventions (McCreanor et al., 2013).

See the paper by Moreno (2019) commissioned for this study for further detail on adolescent health and media.

---

income, ranging from 93 percent of teens from households with an annual income of $30,000 or less to 97 percent among teens from households with an annual income of $75,000 or more (Anderson and Jiang, 2018).

As noted earlier, adolescents are particularly vulnerable to the effects of social media, both positive and negative (Walrave et al., 2016). For example, social media can expose adolescents to unhealthy risk behaviors and portray these behaviors as normative, which may increase the likelihood of their engaging in those behaviors. In addition, social media can magnify existing peer influences on behavior. For instance, adolescents may post photos of themselves drinking alcohol that others interpret as desirable. Furthermore, for teens who are already engaging in unhealthy risk behaviors, social media may provide a way to find and interact with others who share these interests or further normalize these behaviors within a given community (Ahn, 2011). In contrast, given their ubiquity and influence on behavior, social media may also represent an important opportunity for future health promotion efforts.

Spiritual Health

Developmental Milestones and Trajectories

O'Donnell defines spiritual health as having a sense of purpose, love, hope, peace, and charity. In this report and consistent with this definition, spirituality refers not only to one's religious beliefs but also to the morals, values, character development, and goal setting that contribute to a person's identity.

Spirituality and religiosity are perhaps the most well-recognized influences on spiritual health. The way in which adolescents choose to engage in spiritual or religious practices varies widely. Among those youth who identify with a particular religious group, some maintain a minor, often cultural affiliation with a religious institution, while others regularly engage with religious practices at home and in religious institutions (Barry, Nelson, and Abo-Zena, 2018).

In line with the broader definition of spiritual health adopted in this report, adolescence is also characterized by identity formation, a process during which youth explore their environments to better understand how they see themselves fitting into the world. While some youth develop identities that align with those of their families, others may explore other identities and values in seeking to develop a personal identity (Hall, 2018a).

An important part of an adolescent's identity development is the formation of a value system, which strongly influences behaviors, plans for the future, interests, and interpersonal relationships (Levesque, 2018). While value systems were traditionally shaped by religious or institutional values, cultural and technological changes have given today's youth opportunities to learn and explore more diverse ideas and opinions in establishing who they are and what they believe (Berzonsky, 2018).

As they establish these values, adolescents also begin to seek out information that informs their attitudes and beliefs about civic and global issues. At the same time, they often become involved in their community through volunteering, participating in school clubs or community organizations, and voting. This time spent learning and engaging in civic issues helps them focus on their emerging role in society (Allen, Bogard, and Yanisch, 2018).

Social and Environmental Influences on the Development of Spiritual Health

Identity and spiritual development are grounded in interpersonal relationships. How a person expresses his or her identity is strongly based in particular contexts.

Religion and spirituality can help adolescents discover a higher sense of purpose, which is associated with greater psychological well-being, a more unified identity, a greater sense of meaning, and fewer health-compromising behaviors (Burrow and Hill, 2011; Sumner, Burrow, and Hill, 2018). Other research has found that a sense of purpose beyond oneself is related to academic performance and persistence among high school students (Yeager et al., 2014). In addition, studies show that more religious/spiritual adolescents report less depression, anxiety, and other psychiatric concerns compared with their less religious/spiritual peers (Yonker, Schnabelrauch, and DeHaan, 2012).

Families play an important role in the development of spiritual identity, as early engagement in religion and spirituality is often mediated by parents and other close adults (Kim and Esquivel, 2011). Beyond engaging with family in religious or spiritual activities, adolescents may also become more interested in their cultural heritage and question the meaning of their family culture as they begin to form their own cultural identity. In developing this cultural identity, adolescents often express themselves by educating others, participating in cultural activities and social groups, or incorporating cultural pride into their self-presentation (Barry, Nelson, and Abo-Zena, 2018).

In addition to religious organizations, other community venues can serve as important sources for youth's identity and spiritual development. For instance, having a pride center allows lesbian, gay, bisexual, transgender, and queer/questioning (LGBTQ) teens from different neighborhoods or schools to gather in a communal space, share their experiences, and support each other (Higa et al., 2014) (see Box 2-4 for more information about LGBTQ youth). In addition, community centers can hold events specifically oriented toward youth that can facilitate social support around shared interests or aspects of identity.

Intellectual Health

Developmental Milestones and Trajectories

The final domain of optimal health is intellectual, which encompasses the skills that lead to academic achievements, career achievements, hobbies, and cultural pursuits. During adolescence and into adulthood, the regions

BOX 2-4
LGBTQ Youth

Adolescence is an important developmental period for all youth. For LGBTQ youth, however, adolescence poses several unique challenges as well as opportunities to provide skills and resources for healthy development, particularly with regard to sexual health.

The number of young people in the United States identifying as LGBTQ has grown in recent years. Data from the 2017 Youth Risk Behavior Survey (YRBS) show that at least 8.0 percent of youth identify as bisexual and 2.4 percent as gay or lesbian (Kann et al., 2018). Data suggest that the number of transgender or gender-nonconforming youth is also growing, with 1.8–3 percent of youth identifying as transgender (Kann et al., 2018; Rider et al., 2018).

Despite increases in the acceptance of LGBTQ persons and the growing number of people who identify as LGBTQ, LGBTQ youth still face substantial health challenges. LGBTQ adolescents continue to be more likely to report victimization, both at school and in their homes, compared with adolescents who are heterosexual and cisgender (those whose gender identity aligns with their sex assigned at birth (Austin, Herrick, and Proescholdbell, 2016; McKay, Lindquist, and Misra, 2017; Russell et al., 2014; Toomey and Russell, 2016). High rates of harassment and victimization contribute to the consistent findings of research that, compared with their heterosexual peers, LGBTQ youth are more likely to report depression, alcohol and tobacco use, and sexually transmitted infections and adolescent pregnancy (Goldbach et al., 2014; Hall, 2018b; Saewyc, 2014; Tornello, Riskind, and Patterson, 2014).

Increasingly, researchers have demonstrated that there are pathways that promote resilience and healthy development among LGBTQ youth. For example, facilitating healthy parent–child relationships and parents' acceptance of their LGBTQ children provides a powerful protective factor for LGBTQ youth, being associated with greater self-esteem, social support, lower rates of substance abuse, and improved mental health (Ryan et al., 2010). Schools are also an important venue for promoting resilience among LGBTQ adolescents. LGBTQ students in schools with gay–straight alliances and other policies that prohibit LGBTQ-based bullying report higher levels of classmate and teacher support and less bullying (Day et al., 2019). In addition, policies that allow transgender students to use the bathroom of their choice in schools have been linked to lower levels of sexual assault of transgender students, and LGBTQ-inclusive sexual education is associated with lower rates of bullying, depression, substance use, and sexual risk-taking behaviors among not only LGBTQ students, but also their heterosexual peers (Anderson and Jiang, 2018; Baams, Dubas, and van Aken, 2017; Day et al., 2019; Kull et al., 2016; Murchison et al., 2019; Proulx et al., 2019).

See the paper by Everett (2019) commissioned for this study for further detail on LGBTQ youth.

of the brain that regulate executive functioning and oversee critical abilities for decision making gradually develop (Giedd, 2015; Johnson, Blum, and Giedd, 2009). In addition, improved abstract thinking allows youth to process information, use evidence to draw conclusions, and engage in strategic problem solving and deductive reasoning (Kuhn, 2009).

Social and Environmental Influences on the Development of Intellectual Health

While the school environment itself has perhaps the greatest overall influence on intellectual health, parents, peers, and others also have important impacts in this domain.

Research shows that parenting styles contribute to intellectual health outcomes. Compared with other parenting styles, authoritative parenting, characterized by frequent involvement and supervision, is associated with greater academic achievement (Pinquart, 2016). In particular, research shows that parents' engagement and involvement in their children's schools are associated with better academic outcomes (LaRocque, Kleiman, and Darling, 2011). In addition, adolescent perceptions of closeness and trust with their parents predict better academic competence, engagement, and achievement (Murray, 2009).

The adolescent's peer group can also influence academic achievement and identity. Research shows that high-quality peer relationships are associated with academic engagement and achievement, reflecting a desire to be like high-achieving friends or a shared social identity that affects student behaviors (Juvonen, Espinoza, and Knifsend, 2012; Martin and Dowson, 2009).

Dropping out of high school is strongly associated with poor intellectual health, as it can lead to numerous adverse outcomes, including low wages, unemployment, incarceration, and poverty (Wilson et al., 2011). Dropout rates vary by state, ethnic background, and socioeconomic status (Cataldi and KewalRamani, 2009). The National Center for Education Statistics (2019a) reports that Asian/Pacific Islander students had the highest public school graduation rates in 2016–2017 at 91 percent, followed by white students at 89 percent, and significantly lower rates among Hispanic/Latino (80%), black (78%), and American Indian/Alaska Native (72%) students. Generally, males are more likely than females to drop out of high school (National Center for Education Statistics, 2019b). However, teenage pregnancy and parenthood significantly increase the risk of dropout for adolescent girls, with only 50 percent of teenage mothers in the United States earning a high school diploma by age 22 (Perper, Peterson, and Manlove, 2010).

The single greatest predictor of gaps in academic achievement by race and income is the segregation of schools by family income (NASEM, 2019).

Schools in neighborhoods with lower socioeconomic status, where students are more likely to be people of color, typically are less well funded, have less-qualified teachers, and have fewer resources relative to schools in wealthier areas. All of these factors can affect academic outcomes for students. As income inequality continues to rise, so does income segregation among schools, which denies youth from low-income families equal opportunities for success. For this reason, *The Promise of Adolescence* (NASEM, 2019) report emphasizes that children from adverse circumstances need *more* rather than equal resources if society is truly going to reduce disparities in educational outcomes.

Regarding social media, many studies indicate that educators can take advantage of these technology platforms to engage effectively with students, such as by having them complete online courses, tests, or assignments; watch instructional videos; conduct research; and participate virtually in classroom activities, as well as by fostering communication between students and teachers (Ahn, 2011; Greenhow, Sonnevend, and Agur, 2016). Such technology platforms can also help to engage more effectively with students with disabilities (see Box 2-5 for more information about adolescents with disabilities).

As with other aspects of optimal health, however, these technologies can have adverse effects on intellectual health. For example, multitasking on social media may come at the expense of academic work and put youth at higher risk of exposure to inaccurate information. Much attention has been given to the spread of misinformation online, and a 2018 study reported in *Science* found that such misinformation spreads faster than the truth (Vosoughi, Roy, and Aral, 2018). Adolescents are particularly vulnerable in this regard, since their developing cognitive skills may make it more difficult for them to judge information. Promoting digital literacy for adolescents can therefore provide them with the necessary tools to avoid and interpret misinformation.

CONCLUSIONS

This chapter has defined and applied O'Donnell's optimal health framework to the context of normative adolescent development and highlighted how that development is influenced by the physical and social environments. Based on the evidence presented in this chapter, the committee drew the following conclusions.

CONCLUSION 2-1: Adolescents face variations in access to opportunities and supports that often relate to age, race and ethnicity, socioeconomic status, rurality/urbanity, sexual orientation, sex and gender, and disability.

BOX 2-5
Adolescents with Disabilities

Recent decades have seen efforts to distinguish between the constructs of disability and health (Krahn et al., 2009). When these concepts are understood as separate, it follows logically that people with disabilities can be either sick or healthy; thus, one can have a disability and also experience good or excellent health (U.S. Department of Health and Human Services, 2005). Important in this view is the recognition that many of the health problems experienced by people with disabilities are preventable (Krahn et al., 2009). Accordingly, addressing the health needs of individuals with disabilities is an important responsibility of public health, comparable to addressing health disparities experienced by other marginalized groups (Iezzoni, 2011; Krahn et al., 2009).

Approximately 15 percent of children ages 3–17 have a disability (Boyle et al., 2011). The most common causes of disabilities present during the adolescent years are emotional and behavioral disorders, learning disabilities, mild intellectual disability, speech and language impairments, and autism (Gage, Lierheimer, and Goran, 2012). Lower-incidence disabilities in this age range include blindness/low vision, deafness/hard-of-hearing, and physical disabilities (Boyle et al., 2011; Halfon et al., 2012).

Attention to optimal health and improving outcomes of youth with disabilities is greatly needed. Numerous studies have shown that youth with disabilities are more likely to engage in unhealthy risk behaviors and experience adverse outcomes compared with their peers without disabilities. More specifically, youth with disabilities have been shown to be more likely to use alcohol and tobacco and to have unprotected sex and sex with multiple partners. Women with disabilities have also been shown to be less likely to use contraceptive methods, which contributes to higher proportions of unintended pregnancy among those with versus those without disabilities (Bernert, Ding, and Hoban, 2012; Blum, Kelly, and Ireland, 2001; Jones and Lollar, 2008; Mitra et al., 2015; Mosher et al., 2018; Wu et al., 2017).

The dimensions of optimal health are applicable to youth with disabilities in much the same way that they are to youth without disabilities, with some minor variations. Medical self-care is a more central issue for youth with some types of disabilities than it is for those without disabilities, and the focus on medical management of their disability may result in less attention to other aspects of optimal health (Lindsay, 2014). Youth with disabilities may also need greater support in coping with stress and emotional challenges, which may be related to aspects of their disabilities and/or to the social stigma and marginalization they disproportionally experience (Anaby et al., 2013; Kramer et al., 2012; Lindsay, 2014; Tonkin et al., 2014). For similar reasons, attaining and maintaining social health may be more challenging for youth with disabilities. Relationships with family, friends, teachers, and others can therefore serve as crucial buffers against the more negative social interactions that youth with disabilities may encounter (Kramer et al., 2012; Lindsay, 2014; Whitehill, Brockman, and Moreno, 2013).

See the paper by Horner-Johnson and Sauvé (2019) commissioned for this study for further detail on youth with disabilities.

CONCLUSION 2-2: The physical and social environments, including parents and family, peers, schools, neighborhoods, and media, have a major influence on adolescent development and well-being.

CONCLUSION 2-3: Adolescents from disadvantaged backgrounds need more resources relative to their peers from more advantaged backgrounds to ensure their access to comparable opportunities.

The next chapter addresses normative adolescent risk taking and describes the current landscape of adolescent alcohol use, tobacco use, and sexual behavior, as well as their related health outcomes.

REFERENCES

Ahn, J. (2011). The effect of social network sites on adolescents' social and academic development: Current theories and controversies. *Journal of the American Society for Information Science and Technology, 62*(8), 1435–1445.

Allen, L., Bogard, K., and Yanisch, T. (2018). Civic and citizenship attitudes. In R.J.R. Levesque (Ed.), *Encyclopedia of Adolescence* (pp. 600–606). Basel, Switzerland: Springer International.

Allwood, M.A., Baetz, C., DeMarco, S., and Bell, D.J. (2012). Depressive symptoms, including lack of future orientation, as mediators in the relationship between adverse life events and delinquent behaviors. *Journal of Child & Adolescent Trauma, 5*(2), 114–128.

Anaby, D., Hand, C., Bradley, L., DiRezze, B., Forhan, M., DiGiacomo, A., and Law, M. (2013). The effect of the environment on participation of children and youth with disabilities: A scoping review. *Disability and Rehabilitation, 35*(19), 1589–1598.

Anderson, M., and Jiang, J. (2018). *Teens, Social Media & Technology 2018.* Washington, DC: Pew Research Center.

Austin, A., Herrick, H., and Proescholdbell, S. (2016). Adverse childhood experiences related to poor adult health among lesbian, gay, and bisexual individuals. *American Journal of Public Health, 106*(2), 314–320.

Aylwin, C.F., Toro, C.A., Shirtcliff, E., and Lomniczi, A. (2019). Emerging genetic and epigenetic mechanisms underlying pubertal maturation in adolescence. *Journal of Research on Adolescence, 29*(1), 54–79.

Baams, L., Dubas, J.S., and van Aken, M.A.G. (2017). Comprehensive sexuality education as a longitudinal predictor of LGBTQ name-calling and perceived willingness to intervene in school. *Journal of Youth and Adolescence, 46*(5), 931–942.

Bakadorova, O., and Raufelder, D. (2017). The interplay of students' school engagement, school self-concept and motivational relations during adolescence. *Frontiers in Psychology, 8*(2171).

Barry, C.T., Sidoti, C.L., Briggs, S.M., Reiter, S.R., and Lindsey, R.A. (2017). Adolescent social media use and mental health from adolescent and parent perspectives. *Journal of Adolescence, 61*, 1–11.

Barry, C.M., Nelson, L.J., and Abo-Zena, M.M. (2018). Religiousness in adolescence and emerging adulthood. In R.J.R. Levesque (Ed.), *Encyclopedia of Adolescence* (pp. 3101–3126). Basel, Switzerland: Springer International.

Bernert, D.J., Ding, K., and Hoban, M.T. (2012). Sexual and substance use behaviors of college students with disabilities. *American Journal of Health Behavior, 36*(4), 459–471.

Berzonsky, M.D. (2018). Identity processes. In R.J.R. Levesque (Ed.), *Encyclopedia of Adolescence* (pp. 1828–1836). Basel, Switzerland: Springer International.

Blum, R.W., Kelly, A., and Ireland, M. (2001). Health-risk behaviors and protective factors among adolescents with mobility impairments and learning and emotional disabilities. *Journal of Adolescent Health, 28*(6), 481–490.

Bowker, A., and Ramsay, K. (2018). Friendship characteristics. In R.J.R. Levesque (Ed.), *Encyclopedia of Adolescence* (pp. 1487–1494). Basel, Switzerland: Springer International.

Boyle, C.A., Boulet, S., Schieve, L.A., Cohen, R.A., Blumberg, S.J., Yeargin-Allsopp, M., Visser, S., and Kogan, M.D. (2011). Trends in the prevalence of developmental disabilities in U.S. children, 1997–2008. *Pediatrics, 127*(6), 1034–1042.

Boz, N., Uhls, Y.T., and Greenfield, P.M. (2016). Cross-cultural comparison of adolescents' online self-presentation strategies: Turkey and the United States. *International Journal of Cyber Behavior, Psychology and Learning, 6*(3), 1–16.

Branje, S., Laursen, B., and Collins, W.A. (2012). Parent–child communication during adolescence. In A.L. Vangelisti (Ed.), *The Routledge Handbook of Family Communication* (pp. 283–298). New York, NY: Routledge.

Brown, M.B. and Bolen, L.M. (2018). School-based health centers. In R.J.R. Levesque (Ed.), *Encyclopedia of Adolescence* (pp. 2506–2512). Basel, Switzerland: Springer International.

Burrow, A.L. and Hill, P.L. (2011). Purpose as a form of identity capital for positive youth adjustment. *Developmental Psychology, 47*(4), 1196–1206.

Carthy, T., Horesh, N., Apter, A., Edge, M.D., and Gross, J.J. (2010). Emotional reactivity and cognitive regulation in anxious children. *Behavioral Research and Therapy, 48*(5), 384–393.

Casey, B.J. (2015). Beyond simple models of self-control to circuit-based accounts of adolescent behavior. *Annual Review of Psychology, 66*, 295–319.

Cataldi, E.F. and KewalRamani, A. (2009). *High school dropout and completion rates in the United States: 2007 compendium report.* (NCES 2009-064). U.S. Department of Education, Institute of Education Sciences, National Center for Education Statitistics. Washington, DC. Available: http://nces.ed.gov/pubsearch/pubsinfo.asp?pubid=2009064.

Chou, H-T.Z. and Edge, N. (2012). "They are happier and having better lives than I am": The impact of using Facebook on perceptions of others' lives. *Cyberpsychology, Behavior, and Social Networking, 15*(2), 117–121.

Compas, B.E. (2009). Processes of risk and resilience during adolescence. In R.M. Lerner and L. Steinberg (Eds.), *Handbook of Adolescent Psychology* (Vol. 1). Hoboken, NJ: John Wiley & Sons.

Cowie, H. (2019). *From Birth to Sixteen: Children's Health, Social, Emotional and Linguistic Development* (2nd ed.). New York, NY: Routledge.

Dang, M.T., Conger, K.J., Breslau, J., and Miller, E. (2014). Exploring protective factors among homeless youth: The role of natural mentors. *Journal of Health Care for the Poor and Underserved, 25*(3), 1121–1138.

Day, J.K., Fish, J.N., Grossman, A.H., and Russell, S.T. (2019). Gay-straight alliances, inclusive policy, and school climate: LGBTQ youths' experiences of social support and bullying. *Journal of Research on Adolescence*, 1–13.

DeSteno, D., Gross, J.J., and Kubzansky, L. (2013). Affective science and health: The importance of emotion and emotion regulation. *Health Psychology, 32*(5), 474–486.

Dimock, M. (2019). *Defining Generations: Where Millennials End and Generation Z Begins.* Washington, DC: Pew Research Center.

Epstein, J.L. (2011). *School, Family, and Community Partnerships: Preparing Educators and Improving Schools* (2nd ed.). Philadelphia, PA: Westview Press.

Everett, B.G. (2019). Optimal adolescent health to improve behavioral outcomes for LGBTQ youth. *Paper Commissioned by the Committee on Applying Lessons of Optimal Adolescent Health to Improve Behavioral Outcomes for Youth.* Available: https://www.nap.edu/resource/25552/Optimal%20Adolescent%20Health%20to%20Improve%20Behavioral%20Outcomes%20for%20LGBTQ%20Youth.pdf.

Farley, J.P. and Kim-Spoon, J. (2014). The development of adolescent self-regulation: Reviewing the role of parent, peer, friend, and romantic relationships. *Journal of Adolescence, 37*(4), 433–440.

Gage, N.A., Lierheimer, K.S., and Goran, L.G. (2012). Characteristics of students with high-incidence disabilities broadly defined. *Journal of Disability Policy Studies, 23*(3), 168–178.

Giedd, J.N. (2015). The amazing teen brain. *Scientific American, 312*(6), 32–37.

Goldbach, J.T., Tanner-Smith, E.E., Bagwell, M., and Dunlap, S. (2014). Minority stress and substance use in sexual minority adolescents: A meta-analysis. *Prevention Science, 15*(3), 350–363.

Graber, J.A., Nichols, T.R., and Brooks-Gunn, J. (2010). Putting pubertal timing in developmental context: Implications for prevention. *Developmental Psychobiology, 52*(3), 254–262.

Green, J.G., McLaughlin, K.A., Berglund, P.A., Gruber, M.J., Sampson, N.A., Zaslavsky, A.M., and Kessler, R.C. (2010). Childhood adversities and adult psychiatric disorders in the National Comorbidity Survey Replication II: Associations with persistence of DSM-IV disorders. *Archives of General Psychiatry, 67*(2), 124–132.

Greenhow, C., Sonnevend, J., and Agur, C. (2016). *Education and Social Media: Toward a Digital Future.* Cambridge, MA: The MIT Press.

Halfon, N., Houtrow, A., Larson, K., and Newacheck, P.W. (2012). The changing landscape of disability in childhood. *The Future of Children, 22*(1), 13–42.

Hall, S.P. (2018a). Identity status. In R.J.R. Levesque (Ed.), *Encyclopedia of Adolescence* (pp. 1836–1844). Basel, Switzerland: Springer International Publishing.

Hall, W.J. (2018b). Psychosocial risk and protective factors for depression among lesbian, gay, bisexual, and queer youth: A systematic review. *Journal of Homosexuality, 65*(3), 263–316.

Hart, L.M., Cornell, C., Damiano, S.R., and Paxton, S.J. (2015). Parents and prevention: A systematic review of interventions involving parents that aim to prevent body dissatisfaction or eating disorders. *International Journal of Eating Disorders, 48*(2), 157–169.

Herpertz-Dahlmann, B., Bühren, K., and Remschmidt, H. (2013). Growing up is hard: Mental disorders in adolescence. *Deutsches Ärzteblatt International, 110*(25), 432.

Higa, D., Hoppe, M.J., Lindhorst, T., Mincer, S., Beadnell, B., Morrison, D.M., Wells, E.A., Todd, A., and Mountz, S. (2014). Negative and positive factors associated with the well-being of lesbian, gay, bisexual, transgender, queer, and questioning (LGBTQ) youth. *Youth & Society, 46*(5), 663–687.

Hills, A.P., Dengel, D.R., and Lubans, D.R. (2015). Supporting public health priorities: Recommendations for physical education and physical activity promotion in schools. *Progress in Cardiovascular Diseases, 57*(4), 368–374.

Horner-Johnson, W., and Sauvé, L. (2019). *Applying Lessons of Optimal Adolescent Health to Improve Behavioral Outcomes for Youth with Disabilities.* Paper commissioned by the Committee on Applying Lessons of Optimal Adolescent Health to Improve Behavioral Outcomes for Youth. Available: https://www.nap.edu/resource/25552/Applying%20Lessons%20of%20Optimal%20Adolescent%20Health%20to%20Improve%20Behavioral%20Outcomes%20for%20Youth%20with%20Disabilities.pdf.

Hurd, N.M., Wittrup, A., and Zimmerman, M.A. (2018). Role models. In R.J.R. Levesque (Ed.), *Encyclopedia of Adolescence* (pp. 3179–3186). Basel, Switzerland: Springer International.

Iezzoni, L.I. (2011). Eliminating health and health care disparities among the growing population of people with disabilities. *Health Affairs, 30*(10), 1947–1954.

Ismail, F.Y., Fatemi, A., and Johnston, M.V. (2017). Cerebral plasticity: Windows of opportunity in the developing brain. *European Journal of Paediatric Neurology, 21*(1), 23–48.

Johnson, S.B., Blum, R.W., and Giedd, J.N. (2009). Adolescent maturity and the brain: The promise and pitfalls of neuroscience research in adolescent health policy. *Journal of Adolescent Health, 45*(3), 216–221.

Jones, S.E., and Lollar, D.J. (2008). Relationship between physical disabilities or long-term health problems and health risk behaviors or conditions among U.S. high school students. *Journal of School Health, 78*(5), 252–257.

Juvonen, J., Espinoza, G., and Knifsend, C. (2012). The role of peer relationships in student academic and extracurricular engagement. In S.L. Christenson, A.L. Reschly, and C. Wylie (Eds.), *Handbook of Research on Student Engagement* (pp. 387–401). Boston, MA: Springer.

Kann, L., McManus, T., Harris, W.A., Shanklin, S.L., Flint, K.H., Queen, B., Lowry, R., Chyen, D., Whittle, L., Thornton, J., Lim, C., Bradford, D., Yamakawa, Y., Leon, M., Brener, N., and Ethier, K.A. (2018). Youth risk behavior surveillance—United States, 2017. *Morbidity and Mortality Weekly Report Surveillance Summaries, 67*(8).

Kim, S., and Esquivel, G.B. (2011). Adolescent spirituality and resilience: Theory, research, and educational practices. *Psychology in the Schools, 48*(7), 755–765.

Krahn, G.L., Fujiura, G., Drum, C.E., Cardinal, B.J., and Nosek, M.A. (2009). The dilemma of measuring perceived health status in the context of disability. *Disability and Health Journal, 2*(2), 49–56.

Kramer, J., Olsen, S., Mermelstein, M., Balcells, A., and Liljenquist, K. (2012). Youth with disabilities' perspectives of the environment and participation: A qualitative meta-synthesis. *Child: Care, Health, and Development, 38*(6), 763–777.

Kuhn, D. (2009). Adolescent thinking. In R.M. Lerner and L. Steinberg (Eds.), *Handbook of Adolescent Psychology* (vol. 1, pp. 152–186). Hoboken, NJ: John Wiley & Sons.

Kull, R.M., Greytak, E.A., Kosciw, J.G., and Villenas, C. (2016). Effectiveness of school district antibullying policies in improving LGBT youths' school climate. *Psychology of Sexual Orientation and Gender Diversity, 3*(4), 407–415.

LaRocque, M., Kleiman, I., and Darling, S.M. (2011). Parental involvement: The missing link in school achievement. *Preventing School Failure, 55*(3), 115–122.

Lerner, R.M. and Steinberg, L. (2009). The scientific study of adolescent development: Past, present, and future. In R.M. Lerner and L. Steinberg (Eds.), *Handbook of Adolescent Psychology* (2nd ed., pp. 1–12). Hoboken, NJ: John Wiley & Sons, Inc.

Levesque, R.J.R. (2018). Identity formation. In R.J.R. Levesque (Ed.), *Encyclopedia of Adolescence* (pp. 1826–1828). Basel, Switzerland: Springer International.

Liang, B., Commins, M., and Duffy, N. (2010). Using social media to engage youth: Education, social justice, and humanitarianism. *Prevention Researcher, 17*(5), 13–16.

Lindsay, S. (2014). A qualitative synthesis of adolescents' experiences of living with spina bifida. *Qualitative Health Research, 24*(9), 1298–1309.

Little, K., and Welsh, D. (2018). Romantic experiences. In R.J.R. Levesque (Ed.), *Encyclopedia of Adolescence* (pp. 3186–3194). Basel, Switzerland: Springer International.

Madden, C. (2017). *Hello Gen Z: Engaging the Generation of Post-Millennials*. Sydney, Australia: Hello Clarity.

Martin, A.J., and Dowson, M. (2009). Interpersonal relationships, motivation, engagement, and achievement: Yields for theory, current issues, and educational practice. *Review of Educational Research, 79*(1), 327–365.

McCreanor, T., Lyons, A., Griffin, C., Goodwin, I., Barnes, H.M., and Hutton, F. (2013). Youth drinking cultures, social networking, and alcohol marketing: Implications for public health. *Critical Public Health, 23*(1), 110–120.

McDonald, R.I., Fielding, K.S., and Louis, W.R. (2013). Energizing and de-motivating effects of norm-conflict. *Personality and Social Psychology Bulletin, 39*(1), 57–72.

McElhaney, K.B., and Allen, J.P. (2012). *Sociocultural Perspectives on Adolescent Autonomy* (1st ed.). USA: Oxford University Press.

McKay, T., Lindquist, C.H., and Misra, S. (2017). Understanding (and acting on) 20 years of research on violence and LGBTQ + communities. *Trauma, Violence, & Abuse, 20*(5), 665–678.

McLaughlin, K.A., Hatzenbuehler, M.L., Mennin, D.S., and Nolen-Hoeksema, S. (2011). Emotion dysregulation and adolescent psychopathology: A prospective study. *Behaviour Research and Therapy, 49*(9), 544–554.

McLaughlin, K.A., Green, J.G., Gruber, M.J., Sampson, N.A., Zaslavsky, A.M., and Kessler, R.C. (2012). Childhood adversities and first onset of psychiatric disorders in a national sample of U.S. adolescents. *Archives of General Psychiatry, 69*(11), 1151–1160.

McLaughlin, K.A., Garrad, M.C., and Somerville, L.H. (2015). What develops during emotional development? A component process approach to identifying sources of psychopathology risk in adolescence. *Dialogues in Clinical Neuroscience, 17*(4), 403–410.

Merikangas, K.R., He, J-P., Burstein, M., Swanson, S.A., Avenevoli, S., Cui, L., Benjet, C., Georgiades, K., and Swendsen, J. (2010). Lifetime prevalence of mental disorders in U.S. adolescents: Results from the National Comorbidity Survey Replication–Adolescent supplement (NCS-A). *Journal of the American Academy of Child & Adolescent Psychiatry, 49*(10), 980–989.

Mitra, M., Clements, K.M., Zhang, J., Iezzoni, L.I., Smeltzer, S.C., and Long-Bellil, L.M. (2015). Maternal characteristics, pregnancy complications, and adverse birth outcomes among women with disabilities. *Medical Care, 53*(12), 1027–1032.

Moreno, M.A. (2019). Adolescent health and media. *Paper Commissioned by the Committee on Applying Lessons of Optimal Adolescent Health to Improve Behavioral Outcomes for Youth.* Available: https://www.nap.edu/resource/25552/Adolescent%20Health%20 and%20Media.pdf.

Moreno, M.A., Gower, A.D., Jenkins, M.C., Kerr, B., and Gritton, J. (2018). Marijuana promotions on social media: Adolescents' views on prevention strategies. *Substance Abuse Treatment, Prevention, and Policy, 13*(1), 23.

Mosher, W., Hughes, R.B., Bloom, T., Horton, L., Mojtabai, R., and Alhusen, J.L. (2018). Contraceptive use by disability status: New national estimates from the National Survey of Family Growth. *Contraception, 97*(6), 552–558.

Murchison, G.R., Agénor, M., Reisner, S.L., and Watson, R.J. (2019). School restroom and locker room restrictions and sexual assault risk among transgender youth. *Pediatrics, 143*(6), 1–10.

Murray, C. (2009). Parent and teacher relationships as predictors of school engagement and functioning among low-income urban youth. *Journal of Early Adolescence, 29*(3), 376–404.

MyVoice. (2019). Youth perspectives on being healthy and thriving. *Report Commissioned by the Committee on Applying Lessons of Optimal Adolescent Health to Improve Behavioral Outcomes for Youth.* Available: https://www.nap.edu/resource/25552/ Youth%20Perspectives%20on%20Being%20Healthy%20and%20Thriving.pdf.

National Academies of Sciences, Engineering, and Medicine (NASEM). (2019). *The Promise of Adolescence: Realizing Opportunity for all Youth*. Washington, DC: The National Academies Press.

National Center for Education Statistics. (2019a). *Public High School Graduation Rates: 2016-2017*. Available: https://nces.ed.gov/fastfacts/display.asp?id=805.

National Center for Education Statistics. (2019b). *Dropout Rates*. Available: https://nces.ed.gov/fastfacts/display.asp?id=16.

Nesi, J., Choukas-Bradley, S., and Prinstein, M.J. (2018). Transformation of adolescent peer relations in the social media context: Part 2—application to peer group processes and future directions for research. *Clinical Child and Family Psychology Review, 21*, 295–319.

Noller, P. and Atkin, S. (2014). *Family Life in Adolescence*. Berlin, Germany: Walter de Gruyter GmbH.

O'Donnell, M.P. (1986). Definition of health promotion. *American Journal of Health Promotion, 1*(1), 4–5.

O'Donnell, M.P. (2009). Definition of health promotion 2.0: Embracing passion, enhancing motivation, recognizing dynamic balance, and creating opportunities. *American Journal of Health Promotion, 24*(1), iv.

O'Donnell, M.P. (2017). *Health Promotion in the Workplace* (5th ed.). Troy, MI: Art & Science of Health Promotion Institute.

Parasuraman, S.R., and Shi, L. (2014). The role of school-based health centers in increasing universal and targeted delivery of primary and preventive care among adolescents. *Journal of School Health, 84*(8), 524–532.

Parent, A-S., Franssen, D., Fudvoye, J., Pinson, A., and Bourguignon, J-P. (2016). Current changes in pubertal timing: Revised vision in relation with environmental factors including endocrine disruptors. *Puberty from Bench to Clinic, 29*, 174–184. Basel, Switzerland: Karger Publishers.

Perper, K., Peterson, K., and Manlove, J. (2010). Diploma attainment among teen mothers. Fact Sheet. *Child Trends, 2010-01*.

Pinquart, M. (2016). Associations of parenting styles and dimensions with academic achievement in children and adolescents: A meta-analysis. *Educational Psychology Review, 28*(3), 475–493.

Proulx, C.N., Coulter, R.W.S., Egan, J.E., Matthews, D.D., and Mair, C. (2019). Associations of lesbian, gay, bisexual, transgender, and questioning–inclusive sex education with mental health outcomes and school-based victimization in U.S. high school students. *Journal of Adolescent Health, 64*(5), 608–614.

Rider, G.N., McMorris, B.J., Gower, A.L., Coleman, E., and Eisenberg, M.E. (2018). Health and care utilization of transgender and gender nonconforming youth: A population-based study. *Pediatrics, 141*(3), e20171683.

Russell, S.T., Everett, B.G., Rosario, M., and Birkett, M. (2014). Indicators of victimization and sexual orientation among adolescents: Analyses from youth risk behavior surveys. *American Journal of Public Health, 104*(2), 255–261.

Ryan, C., Russell, S.T., Huebner, D., Diaz, R., and Sanchez, J. (2010). Family acceptance in adolescence and the health of LGBT young adults. *Journal of Child and Adolescent Psychiatric Nursing, 23*(4), 205–213.

Saewyc, E.M. (2014). Adolescent pregnancy among lesbian, gay, and bisexual teens. In A.L. Cherry and M.E. Dillon (Eds.), *International Handbook of Adolescent Pregnancy: Medical, Psychosocial, and Public Health Responses* (pp. 159–169). Boston, MA: Springer U.S.

Seemiller, C., and Grace, M. (2018). *Generation Z: A Century in the Making*. Abingdon, UK: Routledge.

Selemon, L.D. (2013). A role for synaptic plasticity in the adolescent development of executive function. *Translational Psychiatry, 3*, e238.

Smetana, J.G., Robinson, J., and Rote, W.M. (2015). Socialization in adolescence. *Handbook of Socialization: Theory and Research*, 60–84.

Smokowski, P.R., and Evans, C.B.R. (2019). *Bullying and Victimization Across the Lifespan: Playground Politics and Power*. Cham: Switzerland: Springer.

Steinberg, L. (2014). *Age of Opportunity: Lessons from the New Science of Adolescence*. Boston, MA: Houghton Mifflin Harcourt.

Sumner, R., Burrow, A.L., and Hill, P.L. (2018). The development of purpose in life among adolescents who experience marginalization: Potential opportunities and obstacles. *American Psychologist, 73*(6), 740–752.

Thompson, A.E., Greeson, J.K.P., and Brunsink, A.M.. (2016). Natural mentoring among older youth in and aging out of foster care: A systematic review. *Children and Youth Services Review, 61*, 40–50.

Thompson, R.S.Y., and Leadbeater, B.J. (2013). Peer victimization and internalizing symptoms from adolescence into young adulthood: Building strength through emotional support. *Journal of Research on Adolescence, 23*(2), 290–303.

Tonkin, B.L., Ogilvie, B.D., Greenwood, S.A., Law, M.C., and Anaby, D.R. (2014). The participation of children and youth with disabilities in activities outside of school: A scoping review. *Canadian Journal of Occupational Therapy, 81*(4), 226–236.

Toomey, R.B. and Russell, S.T. (2016). The role of sexual orientation in school-based victimization: A meta-analysis. *Youth & Society, 48*(2), 176–201.

Tornello, S.L., Riskind, R.G., and Patterson, C.J. (2014). Sexual orientation and sexual and reproductive health among adolescent young women in the United States. *Journal of Adolescent Health, 54*(2), 160–168.

U.S. Department of Health and Human Services. (2005). *The Surgeon General's Call to Action to Improve the Health and Wellness of Persons with Disabilities*. Rockville, MD: U.S. Department of Health and Human Services, Office of the Surgeon General.

Viner, R.M., Ozer, E.M., Denny, S., Marmot, M., Resnick, M., Fatusi, A., and Currie, C. (2012). Adolescence and the social determinants of health. *The Lancet, 379*(9826), 1641–1652.

Vosoughi, S., Roy, D., and Aral, S. (2018). The spread of true and false news online. *Science, 359*(6380), 1146–1151.

Walker, S.C., Kerns, S.E.U., Lyon, A.R., Bruns, E.J., and Cosgrove, T.J. (2010). Impact of school-based health center use on academic outcomes. *Journal of Adolescent Health, 46*(3), 251–257.

Walrave, M., Ponnet, K., Vanderhoven, E., Haers, J., and Segaert, B. (2016). *Youth 2.0: Social Media and Adolescence*. New York, NY: Springer.

Wang, M-T., and Eccles, J.S. (2013). School context, achievement motivation, and academic engagement: A longitudinal study of school engagement using a multidimensional perspective. *Learning and Instruction, 28*, 12–23.

Whitehill, J.M., Brockman, L.N., and Moreno, M.A. (2013). "Just talk to me": Communicating with college students about depression disclosures on Facebook. *Journal of Adolescent Health, 52*(1), 122–127.

Wilson, S.J., Tanner-Smith, E.E., Lipsey, M.W., Steinka-Fry, K., and Morrison, J. (2011). Dropout prevention and intervention programs: Effects on school completion and dropout among school aged children and youth. *Campbell Systematic Reviews, 8*, 61.

Wong, C.A., Merchant, R.M., and Moreno, M.A. (2014). Using social media to engage adolescents and young adults with their health. *Healthcare, 2*(4), 220–224.

Wu, J.P., McKee, K.S., McKee, M.M., Meade, M.A., Plegue, M.A., and Sen, A. (2017). Use of reversible contraceptive methods among U.S. women with physical or sensory disabilities. *Perspectives on Sexual and Reproductive Health, 49*(3), 141–147.

Yeager, D.S., Henderson, M.D., D'Mello, S., Paunesku, D., Walton, G.M., Spitzer, B.J., and Duckworth, A.L. (2014). Boring but important: A self-transcendent purpose for learning fosters academic self-regulation. *Journal of Personality and Social Psychology, 107*(4), 559–580.

Yonker, J.E., Schnabelrauch, C.A., and DeHaan, L.G. (2012). The relationship between spirituality and religiosity on psychological outcomes in adolescents and emerging adults: A meta-analytic review. *Journal of Adolescence, 35*(2), 299–314.

Zimmerman, M.A., Stoddard, S.A., Eisman, A.B., Caldwell, C.H., Aiyer, S.M., and Miller, A. (2013). Adolescent resilience: Promotive factors that inform prevention. *Child Development Perspectives, 7*(4), 215–220.

3

The Current Landscape of Adolescent Risk Behavior

Living my best life means to be happy and accepting of myself in all aspects. I'm free to make my own decisions and whether they turn out good or bad I know I'm one step closer to where I need to b [*sic*] in life.

Female, age 17[1]

Adolescence has long been considered a period when people are especially susceptible to engaging in risky behaviors. This chapter first examines the nature of adolescent risk taking. It then turns to the three behaviors that the committee selected for targeted inclusion in this report—alcohol use, tobacco use, and sexual behaviors—and their related health outcomes.

As described in Chapter 1, the committee limited itself to three specific behaviors for this report given the limited time frame for the study. In general, these selections were based on (1) the prevalence of these behaviors among today's adolescents, (2) the significant amount of data describing their demographic trends, and (3) the large number of peer-reviewed studies of evidence-based programs that have targeted these behaviors and outcomes. We selected sexual behavior because of the focus in the statement of task on the Teen Pregnancy Prevention (TPP) program; alcohol use because, like sexual behavior, it generally becomes socially acceptable or appropri-

---

[1]Response to MyVoice survey question: "Describe what it would look like to live your best life." See the discussion of the MyVoice methodology in Appendix B for more detail.

ate once a person reaches a particular age or developmental milestone; and tobacco use, because of the decades of research on primary and secondary prevention programs and interventions for nicotine addiction and tobacco-related diseases, which we believed would be informative to our task. We recognize, of course, that selecting only three behaviors resulted in excluding a number of highly prevalent risk behaviors from our in-depth review. We found this to be a particularly difficult decision with regard to violence, which encompasses a set of risk behaviors that are associated with some of the most common causes of morbidity and mortality among adolescents (Centers for Disease Control and Prevention [CDC], 2019a) (see Box 3-1). It is also important to note that violent behaviors often co-occur with the three risk behaviors that are covered in this report. For example, violence in the form of bullying can lead to increased substance use behaviors, and sexual behavior under the influence of alcohol may result in violence in the form of sexual assault. We therefore highlight these connections between violence and our three focal behaviors where relevant.

THE NATURE OF ADOLESCENT RISK TAKING

Risk behavior tends to follow a typical trajectory: it is low in childhood, increases around puberty, peaks in late adolescence to early adulthood, and then decreases in adulthood (Romer, Reyna, and Satterthwaite, 2017). Researchers posit that risky adolescent behaviors reflect a gap between an adolescent's biological and social maturity. Many studies have also found that adolescents' decision-making processes differ in significant ways from those of adults. First, adolescents often underestimate risks and perceive greater potential benefits from risky behavior (Smith, Chein, and Steinberg, 2014). Second, while adults avoid risky behavior by engaging in gist-based reasoning (defined as reasoning based on intuitive reactions derived from education and experiences), adolescents lack the experience to employ such reasoning (Reyna, 2012). Third, adolescents use emotion-based reasoning, meaning that rather than just weighing the risks, they also think about the social consequences of their decisions (Blakemore and Robbins, 2012). Finally, when adolescents do engage in risky behaviors, they often have a limited understanding of the possible consequences of their actions (van den Bos and Hertwig, 2017).

Healthy Adolescent Risk Taking

Risk is a general construct that is not confined to illicit or unsafe behaviors. Healthy risk taking involves socially acceptable and constructive risk behaviors, and as discussed previously, is considered a necessary and normative part of adolescence (Duell and Steinberg, 2019). These behaviors

---

BOX 3-1
How Violence Relates to This Report

The adolescent risk behaviors that we selected for inclusion in this report are not an exhaustive list. In particular, we recognize that many forms of violence perpetration and victimization, including the use of firearms and other weapons, suicide attempts, bullying, cyberbullying, and dating violence, are prevalent and pervasive in the lives of today's youth (CDC, 2019a).

It is quite difficult for all young people living in the United States not to be impacted by the violence that surrounds them, whether personally or through media exposure. Violent behaviors not only threaten feelings of safety, but also can lead to a number of negative health outcomes, including injury, death by homicide or suicide, and psychological harm. Violence accounts for a large proportion of deaths among adolescents ages 10–19, and also leads to significant morbidity in the form of nonfatal violent injuries and psychosocial issues, including depression, anxiety, and posttraumatic stress disorder (Curtin et al., 2018). Furthermore, the psychological effects of violence that may occur in families and communities can leave adolescents significantly traumatized, fearful, and/or desensitized (CDC, 2019a).

Although it is not one of our three focal behaviors, violence is frequently cited in this report because of its impact on the social environment, particularly for marginalized groups, and its interrelatedness with substance use and sexual behavior. This interrelatedness also extends to prevention programming: establishing safe, inclusive, and equitable environments; engaging families and communities; and promoting social-emotional skills can improve outcomes in all of the areas on which this report focuses, thus helping young people thrive (David-Ferdon et al., 2016).

For more information on violence and violence prevention, see the following relevant National Academies of Sciences, Engineering, and Medicine publications:

- *The Science of Adolescent Risk-Taking: Workshop Report* (Institute of Medicine, 2011)
- *Priorities for Research to Reduce the Threat of Firearm-Related Violence* (Institute of Medicine and National Research Council, 2013)
- *The Evidence for Violence Prevention Across the Lifespan and Around the World: Workshop Summary* (Institute of Medicine and National Research Council, 2014)
- *Preventing Bullying through Science, Policy, and Practice* (NASEM, 2016)
- *Community Violence as a Population Health Issue: Proceedings of a Workshop* (NASEM, 2017)
- *Violence and Mental Health: Opportunities for Prevention and Early Detection: Proceedings of a Workshop* (NASEM, 2018a)

are risky because of the uncertainty of their potential outcomes rather than the severity of their potential costs, and engaging in healthy risk taking allows adolescents to learn, grow, and thrive.

Researchers also refer to healthy risk taking as safe, positive, prosocial, or adaptive risk taking (Duell and Steinberg, 2019; Wood, Dawe, and Gullo, 2013). Such risk taking allows adolescents to explore and become more autonomous. Taking risks also enables adolescents to challenge the values, morals, and beliefs they were taught in order to develop their own identities separate from those of their parents, families, and peers. In addition, healthy risk taking gives adolescents the chance to practice making decisions; test out their new problem-solving skills; and develop realistic assessments of themselves, other people, and the world around them. In all five dimensions of optimal health discussed in Chapter 2 (O'Donnell, 2017), some degree of risk taking is necessary to promote positive health outcomes and prepare for adulthood (Duell and Steinberg, 2019).

Duell and Steinberg (2019) propose three features that characterize healthy risks. First, healthy risks benefit adolescents' well-being. Second, they carry mild potential costs compared with unhealthy risks. And third, they are generally socially acceptable. In this context, social acceptability refers to the views of adults rather than those of other adolescents; although the social acceptability of certain healthy risks may be controversial among adults, social acceptability in adolescence is often more strongly associated with peer culture and contextual influences.

The following are examples of healthy risk taking within each of the five dimensions of optimal health:

1. Physical
   — Participating in a team sport
   — Trying a new food
2. Emotional
   — Reaching out for help
   — Apologizing for a mistake
3. Social
   — Public speaking
   — Asking someone out on a date
4. Intellectual
   — Enrolling in a challenging course
   — Applying knowledge to a new situation
5. Spiritual
   — Experimenting with different values systems and identities
   — Volunteering for a good cause

Unhealthy Adolescent Risk Taking

In contrast to healthy risk taking, unhealthy risk taking encompasses behaviors that can result in adverse consequences that outweigh the potential gains and may delay or harm adolescents' development. From childhood to adolescence, a significant increase occurs in such unhealthy risk-taking behaviors as substance abuse, smoking, violence, and unprotected sexual activity (Institute of Medicine, 2011). Not all adolescents engage in these behaviors often, although many experiment with them. Generally, research has found that serious problems tend to cluster in a small percentage of youth (Cross, Lotfipour, and Leslie, 2017). In addition, adolescents at highest risk for negative consequences often engage in multiple unhealthy risk behaviors, such as drug or alcohol use and unprotected sexual intercourse (Wu et al., 2010).

The following are examples of unhealthy adolescent risk taking within each of the five dimensions of optimal health:

1. Physical
   — Driving under the influence of alcohol
   — Engaging in sexual intercourse without protection
2. Emotional
   — Using coercion
   — Lying
3. Social
   — Provoking a physical fight
   — Bullying or cyberbullying
4. Intellectual
   — Cheating on a test
   — Skipping school
5. Spiritual
   — Engaging in behaviors that go against one's ethical code
   — Doing something because of peer pressure rather than personal beliefs

Characteristics of Adolescent Risk Taking

Although scientists have yet to reach consensus on what exactly drives adolescent risk taking, most agree on certain key components of adolescent risk behavior, including impulsivity, sensation seeking, self-regulation/impulse control, working memory, and response inhibition (Hartley and Somerville, 2015; Roditis et al., 2016).

Some of the most unhealthy adolescent risk behaviors are linked to impulsive traits that appear in early childhood. Higher levels of *impulsivity* in children as early as age 3 have been associated with drug use and aggressive behavior in adolescence (Romer, 2010). Similarly, *sensation seeking,* or the tendency to seek out new or thrilling experiences, can also lead to increased unhealthy risk-taking behavior (Duell and Steinberg, 2019).

Self-regulation, also termed *impulse control,* denotes the process through which individuals effectively handle impulsivity and sensation seeking. Higher self-regulation is associated with fewer unhealthy risk-taking behaviors, including substance use and antisocial behavior, among middle school students (Fosco et al., 2013). Furthermore, research suggests that self-regulation skills can be improved by engaging in positive risk behaviors that require planning and impulse control (Wood, Dawe, and Gullo, 2013). Taken together, these findings indicate that healthy risk taking can provide adolescents with important opportunities to practice self-regulatory skills, and thus narrow the developmental gap between sensation seeking and self-regulation during adolescence.

Another component of adolescent risk behavior is *working memory,* or the capacity to temporarily store and manipulate a limited quantity of goal-relevant information in order to perform complex cognitive tasks (Murty, Calabro, and Luna, 2016). Working memory supports more goal-oriented versus impulsive actions because adolescents can use past risk-taking experiences to inform future behavior (Hofmann, Schmeichel, and Baddeley, 2012; Romer, Reyna, and Satterthwaite, 2017). In contrast, adolescents with worse working memory may be more likely to engage in unhealthy risk-taking behavior and may be less likely to incorporate learning from past experiences into their decision-making processes.

Strongly related to working memory, *response inhibition* is the capacity to suppress a behavioral response in favor of one that is more appropriate or goal oriented. Research has found that lower response inhibition in adolescents is related to more unhealthy risk behaviors, including unsafe driving, early cigarette smoking, and alcohol use (Henges and Marczinski, 2012; Mashhoon et al., 2018; Ross et al., 2015).

Ultimately, adolescent risk-taking behavior is influenced by many complex and interacting variables, including aspects of brain development and biological processes, as well as proximal and distal contextual factors. In general, most theorists agree that risk taking during adolescence is normal, but that the key to healthy risk taking is to provide guidance in decision making and to encourage adolescents to engage in less dangerous and more constructive risks.

Neurobiological Factors in Adolescent Risk Taking

Advances in understanding of human brain development have yielded insights into why adolescents may be more predisposed to unhealthy risk taking relative to children or adults (Graber, Nichols, and Brooks-Gunn, 2010). At the onset of puberty, adolescent boys produce more testosterone, a hormone associated with sensation seeking and aggressive risk taking. For girls, increased testosterone is associated with the tendency to affiliate with peers who engage in unhealthy risk behaviors (Vermeersch et al., 2008). In line with more comprehensive, whole-brain approaches, neuroscientists have begun to investigate how increases in these gonadal hormones at puberty may contribute to risk-taking behaviors during adolescence by altering neural responses to rewards (Braams et al., 2015).

The hormonal changes that occur during puberty remodel the socio-emotional network in the limbic and paralimbic areas of the brain. This network, which is particularly important for thrill seeking and sensitivity to rewards, develops more quickly and is more active during adolescence than during childhood or adulthood. In contrast, the cognitive-control network, which engages the prefrontal cortex, develops more slowly and continues to mature over the course of adolescence and into young adulthood. Studies have found that the competitive dynamic between these two networks is associated with numerous decision-making contexts, including drug use, social decision processing, moral judgments, and the valuation of alternative rewards and costs (Smith, Chein, and Steinberg, 2013).

Context Matters: Social and Environmental Influences on Risk Taking

While there are some developmental constants in terms of the neuro-cognitive and hormonal changes that take place during adolescence, these biological changes occur in the broader socioecological contexts of the parents and family, peer groups, school, and the community (Bronfenbrenner, 1994). The following sections explore these contexts and how they can serve as either risk or protective factors. Many of these contexts are also highlighted in the youth perspectives in Box 3-2.

Individual Influences

Beyond the neurobiological developments that occur during adolescence, individual factors can protect against unhealthy risk taking. These include engagement in meaningful activities, life skills and social competence, positive personal traits, and future orientation (Judd, 2019). *Meaningful activities* promote positive development, including the development of important skills. *Life skills and social competence*—encompassing social-emotional skills related to self-awareness, self-management, social awareness, and communication—help adolescents make positive choices, maintain healthy relationships, and promote their own well-being. *Positive personal traits* that are protective against unhealthy risk behaviors include

BOX 3-2
Youth Voices:
What, if anything, keeps you from living your best life?

In a recent MyVoice survey, adolescents were asked what, if anything, keeps them from living their best life (see Appendix B for more detail on the MyVoice methodology). The top 10 answers and illustrative quotes from the 867 respondents are shown in the figure below. Overall, youth overwhelmingly noted a lack of money as holding them back, along with their own bad habits, behaviors, or self-doubt.

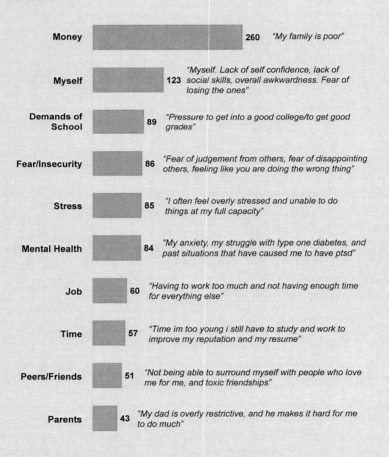

Money	260	"My family is poor"
Myself	123	"Myself. Lack of self confidence, lack of social skills, overall awkwardness. Fear of losing the ones"
Demands of School	89	"Pressure to get into a good college/to get good grades"
Fear/Insecurity	86	"Fear of judgement from others, fear of disappointing others, feeling like you are doing the wrong thing"
Stress	85	"I often feel overly stressed and unable to do things at my full capacity"
Mental Health	84	"My anxiety, my struggle with type one diabetes, and past situations that have caused me to have ptsd"
Job	60	"Having to work too much and not having enough time for everything else"
Time	57	"Time im too young i still have to study and work to improve my reputation and my resume"
Peers/Friends	51	"Not being able to surround myself with people who love me for me, and toxic friendships"
Parents	43	"My dad is overly restrictive, and he makes it hard for me to do much"

SOURCE: Generated using data from the MyVoice (2019) report.

an easy-going temperament, a sense of purpose, and a feeling of control over one's environment. And *future orientation*, or the ability to set future plans or goals, can also protect adolescents against unhealthy risk taking by making them more strategic in choosing risks that have the most potential benefit while posing the least threat to their future plans (Maslowsky et al., 2019).

Parent and Family Influences

A large proportion of U.S. children spend at least some part of their childhood or adolescence in a single-parent family, and an increasing number live with cohabiting, unmarried parents (Livingston, 2018). Generally, research suggests that adolescents who live in single-parent families are more likely to engage in unhealthy risk behaviors and fare worse on a wide range of developmental outcomes relative to their counterparts in families with two biological parents (Langton and Berger, 2011).

Adolescents model their own behavior on that of their family members, peers, and role models. Parents' own risk-taking behavior therefore factors strongly into how adolescents engage with risky activities, which can be related to genetics and to aspects of early learning about substance use (Smit et al., 2018). In addition, exposure to various forms of stress during childhood is associated with later unhealthy risk taking (Institute of Medicine, 2011). Early stressors in the household, including physical and emotional abuse, emotional neglect, parental substance use, and exposure to family violence, are associated with poor health outcomes during adolescence, including drug use, addiction, and suicide. Adolescents who experience such stressors in childhood also tend to have more difficulty with emotion regulation, response inhibition, and executive functioning, and are more likely to fail school, to be excluded from prosocial groups, and to associate with peers who engage in substance use (Romer, 2010).

Parents are often faced with difficult decisions as their children enter adolescence, as adolescents' increasing autonomy from their parents and greater propensity for unhealthy risk taking requires a balance of both trust and behavioral monitoring. Parenting styles characterized by setting high expectations for behavior, establishing clear family rules, applying fair and consistent discipline, and engaging in age-appropriate supervision and monitoring can be protective against unhealthy risk-taking behaviors (Judd, 2019).

As discussed in Chapter 2, adolescents frequently drift away from their parents and toward peer groups. Yet despite this trend, parents continue to play an important role in adolescents' lives, although the changing nature of these relationships can have significant effects on risk taking and associated health outcomes (Tsai, Telzer, and Fuligni, 2013). Family connectedness, which refers to feelings of warmth, love, caring, and communication, is also a major protective factor against adolescent risk taking. Adolescents who feel family support and connection report a high degree of closeness with their parents and feelings of being understood, loved, and wanted (Sieving et al., 2017).

Peer Influences

Increasing involvement with peers is one of the primary features distinguishing adolescence from childhood. Research suggests that there are four modes of direct or indirect peer influence, which can operate independently or concurrently: (1) direct peer pressure, (2) peer influence through modeling, (3) influences through group norms, and (4) the creation of structured opportunities (Goliath and Pretorius, 2016; McWhirter et al., 2013).

Numerous studies have shown that, in the presence of peers, adolescents prefer more immediate rewards and engage in more risky behaviors even when they are presented with the potential harms (Knoll et al., 2015; Smith, Chein, and Steinberg, 2014). In addition to peer influence, adolescent peer groups congregate in new, often unsupervised contexts that can facilitate risk-taking behaviors (Institute of Medicine, 2011).

Peers also serve as adolescents' primary source of information about social norms. Peers socialize one another to norms in two ways: by modeling behavior and by reinforcing behavior in other people (Albert, Chein, and Steinberg, 2013). This influence can have both positive and negative effects on risk taking. For instance, teenagers who believe that their peers disapprove of having sex are less likely to become sexually active, whereas teenagers who believe their peers are having sex are more likely to become sexually active (Warner et al., 2011).

In a similar vein, risk taking also relates to the traits adolescents seek in their friends. For instance, adolescents prone to sensation seeking often gravitate toward peers with the same interests. Likewise, adolescents who lack social skills or social competence may incur a negative reputation, which may lead them to peers who share the same deficits and reinforce negative social pressures (Institute of Medicine, 2011).

Peer conflict and exclusion are also associated with increased unhealthy risk-taking behavior (Falk et al., 2014; Peake et al., 2013; Telzer et al., 2015). Blakemore (2018) suggests that because adolescents are fundamentally motivated to prevent social rejection by their peers, they may engage in unhealthy risk behaviors that have adverse health or disciplinary consequences. Adolescents may therefore seek and engage in behaviors that adults view as unhealthy risks in order to win peer approval, or at the very least to avoid peer rejection (Maslowsky et al., 2019).

School Influences

School connectedness, which refers to adolescents' beliefs that adults and peers in the school care about them, is an important protective factor for a range of risk behaviors, including early sexual initiation; alcohol, tobacco, and other drug use; and violence (CDC, 2018a). Schools can foster school connectedness by establishing positive norms, providing clear expectations for behavior, and fostering physical and psychological safety for all students (Thapa et al., 2013).

Another important protective factor is positive school climate, which refers to whether adolescents feel that the school environment promotes and encourages connectedness and support. Characteristics of a positive school climate include having high expectations for student academics, behavior, and responsibility; using proactive classroom management strategies; employing interactive teaching and cooperative learning styles; consistently acknowledging all students and recognizing good work; and allowing students to express themselves in school activities and class management (Judd, 2019).

Adolescents need opportunities to engage as learners, leaders, team members, and workers. For this reason, in-school or after-school programs can offer healthy alternatives to unhealthy risk behavior. In addition, such programs and interventions delivered in and after school may be specifically oriented toward the prevention or reduction of unhealthy risk taking, as in the case of drug prevention and sexual education (CDC, 2018a).

Youth–adult connectedness is also essential for adolescent health and well-being. Teachers and coaches can have important influences on adolescents' goals, which are strongly associated with risk-taking behavior. Research shows that close, positive relationships with caring adults outside of the family can protect adolescents from a range of poor health outcomes and promote positive youth development (Sieving et al., 2017).

Finally, parental engagement in schools can be protective against unhealthy risk taking. Research has found that it reduces the likelihood that adolescents will engage in such unhealthy risk behaviors as alcohol use, tobacco use, and unprotected sexual activity. In addition, parental engagement is associated with better student behavior, higher academic achievement, and enhanced social skills (CDC, 2018a).

Community Influences

Structural (e.g., poverty) and social (e.g., norms) characteristics of neighborhoods can shape adolescent risk taking (Leventhal, Dupéré, and Brooks-Gunn, 2009). Neighborhood or community risk factors for unhealthy adolescent risk behaviors include the availability of drugs or firearms, extreme poverty, community disorganization, and low neighborhood attachment. On the other hand, neighborhood resources and opportunities can protect against unhealthy risk taking by increasing structures and supports, particularly for at-risk youth (Holmes et al., 2019).

In particular, access to high-quality, teen-friendly health care can reduce, prevent, and mitigate the effects of unhealthy risk behaviors. Adolescents need medical, dental, and behavioral health services with health care providers who respect and understand their particular needs. In addition, health care that is teen-friendly, culturally competent, affordable, convenient, and confidential can promote adolescent autonomy (U.S. Department of Health and Human Services [HHS}, 2018a).

Beyond improving health services, local, state, and federal governments can take additional measures to discourage unhealthy risk behaviors among adolescents. One successful example is graduated driver's licensing laws, which have been associated with a 42 percent reduction in the nationwide rate of crashes involving 16-year-olds (Institute of Medicine, 2011). Accordingly, similar legislative measures, such as raising the minimum age for smoking and drinking and providing free and easier access to contraception, may also help to mitigate unhealthy adolescent risk taking (Catalano et al., 2012).

Technological Influences

The rapid rise of new technologies has vastly expanded the ways in which adolescents interact and spend their time. Social media are one of the primary ways in which teenagers engage with technology. Studies have found that social media can have a substantial influence on adolescents' social norms, as they involve simple, fast, and quantifiable measures of peer endorsement (e.g., "Likes") (Sherman et al., 2016). In addition to social media, teenagers use technology in a variety of other ways, such as texting, gaming, streaming, and recording, all of which can facilitate adolescent risk behaviors. For instance, text messaging while driving is widely recognized as an unhealthy risk behavior, making it difficult to react during a potential crash (Gershon et al., 2017; Lee et al., 2014). In contrast, technology can also facilitate healthy risk taking, as in the case of assistive and interactive digital media and social media platforms, which can help youth learn new information, find and communicate with similar peers, and engage with broader social support networks (O'Dea and Campbell, 2011; O'Keeffe and Clarke-Pearson, 2011; Odom et al., 2015).

ALCOHOL USE, TOBACCO USE, AND SEXUAL BEHAVIOR: TRENDS AND INFLUENCES

As stated in Chapter 1, the committee was charged with identifying the risk behaviors and outcomes to review for this report. This section describes the demographic trends and social and environmental factors associated with the three adolescent risk behaviors selected by the committee—alcohol use, tobacco use, and sexual behavior—as well as their related adverse health outcomes.

Data Sources

Data on health outcomes in this section come from various federal data sources, including the Centers for Disease Control and Prevention's (CDC's) surveillance systems, the U.S. Department of Transportation (DOT), and the National Survey of Family Growth (NSFG). To evaluate trends in risk behavior in the above three areas, we decided to use data from the Youth Risk Behavior Survey (YRBS).

The Youth Risk Behavior Surveillance System (YRBSS) was established in 1990 to monitor the prevalence of a variety of health behaviors among U.S. adolescents that are associated with later morbidity and mortality outcomes (CDC, 2018b). Every 2 years since 1991, the YRBS has been administered to a nationally representative, cross-sectional sample of in-school adolescents in grades 9–12. Approximately 15,000 youth participated in the most recent survey, in 2017, and more than 4.4 million have participated since 1991.

The YRBS has a number of strengths for the purposes of this study. First, it provides information on all three behaviors of interest (alcohol use, tobacco use, and sexual behavior) among the same population of adolescents. None of the other datasets we considered included all of these behaviors. Second, the YRBS has been conducted consistently since 1991, whereas other surveys either lack similar longevity (e.g., the National Youth Tobacco Survey [NYTS]) or may present results from aggregated time intervals (e.g., the NSFG). Finally, a major strength of the YRBS is the way in which items have been updated or added to reflect changing behavior trends (e.g., use of e-cigarettes, cyberbullying) and diverse populations (e.g., LGBTQ youth) (see Figure 3-1).

At the same time, as with all datasets, the YRBS has critical limitations that necessitate caution when interpreting its results for the broader U.S. adolescent population. First and foremost, the YRBS includes only in-school youth. This is a serious limitation when one is examining behavior trends, since research shows that youth who are not in school (e.g., dropped out, incarcerated, homeless) have the highest incidence of risk behaviors and related adverse health outcomes (Edidin et al., 2012; Odgers, Robins, and Russell, 2010; Tolou-Shams et al., 2019). Although the CDC estimates that out-of-school youth represent only 3.4 percent of the adolescent population, recent research using data from the National Center for Education Statistics suggests that this figure could be as high as 10.1 percent

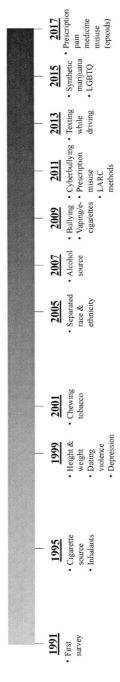

FIGURE 3-1 Items on the Youth Risk Behavior Survey (YRBS) have been updated or added to reflect changes in behaviors and diverse populations over time.

SOURCE: Generated using documentation from the YRBS questionnaires (CDC, 2018c).

(Brener et al., 2013; King, Marino, and Barry, 2018). It is also important to note that the reasons these adolescents are not in school may be related to these risk behaviors. For example, pregnant or parenting teens are more likely to drop out of school (Freudenberg and Ruglis, 2007; Wilson et al., 2011). In addition, substance use or violence in or around school can lead to suspensions, expulsions, and/or juvenile justice involvement (Heitzeg, 2009). Importantly, marginalized youth, particularly adolescents of color, are more likely to experience all of these outcomes (Heitzeg, 2009; Kearney and Levine, 2012).[2]

Similarly, the context in which surveys are administered can affect how participants respond. There is conflicting evidence in the literature regarding the ideal survey setting and mode for asking sensitive behavior questions of adolescents. For example, a study conducted by the CDC in 2004 examined differences in YRBS behavior prevalence estimates by setting (school vs. home) and mode (paper-and-pencil instrument [PAPI] or computer-assisted self-interview [CASI]) (Brener et al., 2006). Results showed that for the majority of YRBS items, including questions about alcohol use and sexual behavior, students who completed the survey in school were more likely to report sensitive behaviors than were those who completed the survey at home. There were fewer differences by survey administration mode; however, those in the CASI condition were more likely to report lifetime alcohol use, current alcohol use, and cigarette smoking before age 13 compared with those in the PAPI condition. Given the relatively few significant differences by mode, the CDC continued using PAPI surveys in school settings because of the relatively greater cost and complexity of CASI administration (Brener et al., 2013).

In 2008, the CDC conducted another study in which students completed the YRBS using (1) a PAPI in school, (2) a Web-based survey in school, or (3) a Web-based survey "on your own" (Eaton et al., 2010). The PAPI and Web-based surveys that were administered in schools showed similar results (Eaton et al., 2010), but more data were missing from the Web-based surveys (Denniston et al., 2010). In addition, the in-school Web-based survey was found to compromise perceived anonymity and both perceived and actual privacy (Denniston et al., 2010). Finally, the response rate was very low among those in the Web-based "on your own" condition (Denniston et al., 2010; Eaton et al., 2010). As a result, the CDC has continued to administer the YRBS in schools using the PAPI mode (Brener et al., 2013).

---

[2]Because of limited reporting, we are unable to present data for all health behaviors and outcomes for all racial/ethnic groups. This is the case in particular for smaller racial/ethnic groups, where small sample sizes required data suppression. In addition, racial/ethnic groups are often defined differently across surveys and over time (e.g., Native Hawaiian/Pacific Islander vs. Asian/Pacific Islander), making them more difficult to compare.

However, recent research suggests that a computer-based mode may be more appropriate for contemporary surveys. A 2015 meta-analysis found that computer-based surveys led to increased response rates to questions about sensitive behaviors among both adolescents and adults (Gnambs and Kaspar, 2015). In addition, there was a significant time trend, with computerized surveys yielding lower response rates in the late 1990s and early 2000s but higher response rates in more recent years, a finding that may be attributable to the overall increase in the use of web-based surveys and widespread access to technology (Gnambs and Kaspar, 2015). Accordingly, further research is needed to understand whether the ideal setting and survey mode for the YRBS have changed within the last decade.

It is also important to note that while YRBS questions have been added or changed over time to reflect more current behavior trends and populations, some questions, particularly those related to sexual behavior, are still ambiguous and exclusive of diverse populations. For example, the first question in the sexual behavior section asks respondents whether they have ever had "sexual intercourse" without defining this term (CDC, 2018c). Therefore, youth may interpret this term to include vaginal sex only, or other types of sexual contact as well, including oral and anal sex (Peck et al., 2016; Sanders and Reinisch, 1999). This is a particularly salient limitation for LGBTQ youth, who may not engage in penile–vaginal intercourse.

Moreover, the subsequent sexual behavior questions present sexual intercourse in a heteronormative way. For example, questions about protection and contraceptive methods are written implicitly and explicitly with pregnancy as the targeted outcome (CDC, 2018c). This is a significant limitation of the YRBS for both heterosexual and LGBTQ youth since, like vaginal sex, oral and anal sex can also lead to sexually transmitted infections (STIs). By contrast, the NSFG asks more specific questions about each type of sexual behavior in a similar age group, which (1) allows for greater precision of the prevalence estimates for each behavior, (2) is more inclusive of diverse behaviors and populations, and (3) provides a better understanding of sequences of sexual behavior initiation.[3]

Other caveats to the national YRBS data need to be considered when interpreting the behavior trends presented in this report. First, the YRBS trends presented in this chapter represent only high school students (approximately 14–18 years old). Although the YRBS is conducted with middle school students in certain sites, these data cannot be analyzed to produce nationally representative estimates (Brener et al., 2013). As mentioned in Chapter 1, although the NYTS and the Monitoring the Future (MTF) survey include middle school students, these surveys report only on substance

---

[3]See Appendix C for a table that compares the wording of sexual behavior items in the YRBS and NSFG.

use. However, the national high school YRBS does include items that ask about experiences before age 13 for each of our behaviors of interest, and therefore serve as a proxy for the prevalence of these behaviors during early adolescence in this report.

Additionally, although schools that participate in the national YRBS are generally not permitted to modify the standard 89-item questionnaire,[4] there are two exceptions to this rule (Brener, 2019).[5] First, many states and localities conduct their own YRBS, for which they have the option of modifying the standard questionnaire within certain parameters (Brener et al., 2013). These data are generally presented separately from the national data; however, if a school is selected into both the national sample and a state/local YRBS sample, the survey is conducted only once (Brener, 2019). In these cases, whether the national or state/local questionnaire is used for the national dataset is dependent on whether the survey is administered by the national contractor or a state/local agency (Brener, 2019). In 2017, for example, 16 of the 144 schools participating in the national survey provided data from a modified state/local questionnaire for the national dataset (Brener, 2019). As a result, the national dataset may be missing information on certain behaviors if the state/local surveys excluded the corresponding items.

The second exception to this rule, although much more rare, occurs when a school or state that is selected into the national sampling frame refuses to participate unless the questionnaire is modified (Brener, 2019). In 2017, this occurred when two schools required that the sexual behavior questions be removed from the survey as a condition of their participation (Brener, 2019). In these scenarios, specific items may not have been asked of a large number of students, which could lead to biased results at the national level. As a result of these limitations, the demographic trends presented in this chapter should be interpreted with caution.

Alcohol Use in Adolescence

Trends

According to the 2017 YRBS, 60.4 percent of U.S. high school students have had at least one drink of alcohol on at least 1 day during their life, compared with 86.1 percent in 1991 (Kann et al., 2018). Trends in current alcohol use, defined as any use in the past 30 days, are similar with

---

[4]Five to 11 questions are added to the standard, national YRBS questionnaire each cycle, and these items generally cover topics that are not covered by the priority health-risk behavior categories (e.g., sun protection) (Brener et al., 2013).

[5]Brener, N. (2019). Personal communication.

50.8 percent of students reporting current alcohol use in 1991 compared with 29.8 percent in 2017 (Kann et al., 2018). Furthermore, early adolescent alcohol use (before age 13) decreased by more than one-half, from 32.7 percent in 1991 to 15.5 percent in 2017 (Kann et al., 2018) (see Figure 3-2).

Underage drinking is associated with many adverse health outcomes, including school and social problems, violence, arrest, unintentional injuries, sexual assault, substance use disorders, and death (Harding et al., 2016; National Research Council and Institute of Medicine, 2004). Heavy alcohol use in adolescence is also neurotoxic to the brain. Alcohol misuse is associated with dysfunction in brain regions underlying impulse control, reward processing, and executive function (Adger Jr. and Saha, 2013). In addition, adolescent alcohol use may increase the risk of developing an alcohol use disorder in early adulthood by altering neural functioning related to rewards (Squeglia et al., 2014).

Alcohol use does not vary significantly by biological sex, but it does vary by race and ethnicity (Kann et al., 2018; NASEM, 2019). In 2017, Asian adolescents reported the lowest rates of current alcohol use (12.2%), followed by black/African American (20.8%), Native Hawaiian/Pacific Islander (26.8%), Hispanic/Latino (31.3%), American Indian/Alaska Native (31.8%), and white (32.4%) youth (CDC, 2019b; Kann et al., 2018) (see Figure 3-3).

Early initiation of alcohol use is a risk factor for a number of adverse consequences. Substance use before age 15 is the most significant predictor of substance dependencies and abuse in late adolescence and adulthood (Lopez-Quintero et al., 2011; HHS, 2017a). Additionally, adolescents who start drinking before age 15 are four times more likely to meet criteria for

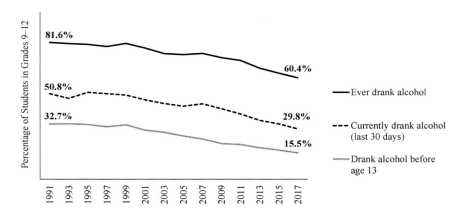

FIGURE 3-2 Adolescent alcohol use has declined since 1991.
SOURCE: Generated using Youth Risk Behavior Survey data (CDC, 2019b).

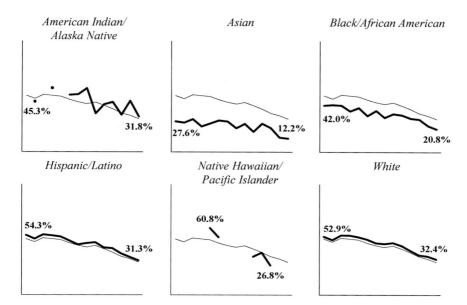

FIGURE 3-3 Percentages of students who currently drink alcohol were lowest among Asians and blacks/African Americans, 1991–2017.
NOTE: Racial/ethnic groups and labels vary by source.
SOURCE: Generated using Youth Risk Behavior Survey data (CDC, 2019b).

alcohol dependence at some point in their lives (HHS, 2017b). However, statistics on early initiation of alcohol are promising. In 2017, 15.5 percent of high school students reported that they had had their first drink of alcohol (other than a few sips) before age 13, compared with 32.7 percent in 1991 (Kann et al., 2018) (see Figure 3-2).

Adolescents who do drink tend to do so less often than adults, yet they are more likely to consume higher quantities of alcohol per occasion (Chung et al., 2018). Underage drinkers ages 12–20 typically consume four to five drinks per occasion, nearly double the average of two to three drinks among adults over age 25 (HHS, 2017a). Binge drinking, defined as having five or more drinks on one occasion for males and four or more drinks on one occasion for females, is the most dangerous way adolescents consume alcohol. Extreme binge drinking is defined as having 10 or more drinks on a single occasion.

The onset of binge drinking and binge drinking episodes typically occurs in early to mid-adolescence (i.e., ages 12–16). Early substance use and rapid progression from first drink to first intoxication are both predictors of binge drinking (Chung, 2018). According to the 2017 YRBS,

13.5 percent of American high school students had engaged in binge drinking during the 30 days before the survey. Nationally, 4.4 percent of students reported that they had consumed 10 or more alcoholic drinks in a row within a couple of hours during the 30 days before the survey. Between 2013 and 2017, there was a noteworthy decrease (6.1% to 4.4%) in the overall prevalence of reporting consumption of 10 or more drinks in a row (Kann et al., 2018).

Substantial research has identified and examined the acute health effects of binge drinking, which include alcohol poisoning, alcohol-related blackouts and injury, car crashes and fatalities, physical and sexual assault, unprotected sexual behavior, and problems at school or work (Hingson and White, 2014; Siqueira and Smith, 2015). The long-term effects of alcohol consumption include an increased risk for heart disease, brain shrinkage, dementia, stroke, liver damage, pancreatitis, lung disease, bone loss, and multiple types of cancer.

Driving under the influence of alcohol is a particular concern with respect to adolescents' alcohol use. Unintentional injuries represent the leading cause of death among adolescents overall,[6] and more than one-half of these deaths result from motor vehicle crashes (CDC, 2019c). The risk is highest among those ages 16–19: in 2017, 2,364 adolescents in this age group died as a result of a motor vehicle crash, and about 300,000 were treated in emergency departments for injuries due to crashes (CDC, 2019d).

Driving under the influence of alcohol and riding with a driver who is under the influence significantly increase the risk of road crashes (Markkula, Härkänen, and Raitasalo, 2019). Drivers are considered to be alcohol impaired when their blood alcohol concentration (BAC) is 0.08 grams per deciliter or greater. Despite declines since 1994, the most recent data from 2017 show that approximately 19 percent of all teen driver fatalities were among those with a BAC over 0.08 g/dl (U.S. Department of Transportation, 2019) (see Figure 3-4).

Social and Environmental Influences

Families play a major role in the development of alcohol-related problems during adolescence. Parental alcohol abuse is a risk factor for adolescent alcohol abuse. Parenting practices including lack of monitoring or supervision of youth, permissive attitudes toward drug use, unclear expec-

---

[6]Although unintentional injury is the overall leading cause of death in the population ages 10–19, this is not true for all racial/ethnic subgroups. In every year since 1999, homicide has represented the leading cause of death among black/African American adolescents, and since 2016, suicide has surpassed unintentional injury as the leading cause of death among Asian/Pacific Islander youth (CDC, 2019c).

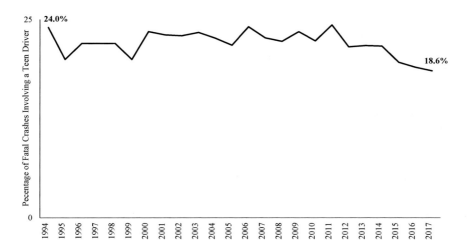

FIGURE 3-4 Proportion of fatal motor vehicle crashes involving a teen driver with a blood alcohol concentration greater than or equal to 0.08 g/dl, 1994–2017.
NOTE: Data from the U.S. Department of Transportation were not disaggregated by biological sex or race/ethnicity.
SOURCE: Generated using data from Young Driver Safety Fact Sheets (U.S. Department of Transportation, 2019).

tations of youth behavior, and no or rare rewarding of positive behavior are also risk factors for the development of substance abuse problems during adolescence (HHS, 2016b).

Equally influential for underage drinking are peer substance use and peer pressure. In particular, selection of peers who engage in binge drinking has been associated with early initiation and increased frequency of substance use (HHS, 2016b). Other social mechanisms that may contribute to high-volume alcohol consumption include peers providing access to alcohol and peer norms that are favorable to binge-drinking behavior (Chung et al., 2018).

Patterns of community use can also predict individual substance use by adolescents. Rates of underage drinking are higher in communities in which alcohol is less expensive and more easily obtainable (HHS, 2016b). Factors associated with where an adolescent chooses to drink, including the level of supervision, privacy, safety, and remoteness, can also impact an adolescent's drinking behavior over time (Chung et al., 2018).

Teenagers are bombarded by positive portrayals of alcohol in the media. Television, movies, and the Internet frequently show alcohol's positive social effects while avoiding its negative effects. Frequent exposure to alcohol advertising, particularly when these advertisements are targeted specifically at teenagers, contributes to social norms around underage drinking (Meisel and Colder, 2019). Furthermore, many studies have shown that media exposure, including portrayals of teenagers drinking on television, can increase adolescents' experimentation with alcohol (Moreno and Whitehill, 2014; Smith and Foxcroft, 2009).

Industry, local, state, and federal alcohol policies also influence adolescent alcohol consumption. In the United States, stronger state alcohol policies and taxes are associated with decreased alcohol consumption among underage youth. In addition, comprehensive and stringent local alcohol control policies and enforcement have been associated with lower levels of youth binge drinking (Paschall, Lipperman-Kreda, and Grube, 2014).

Tobacco Use in Adolescence

Trends

Smoking is the leading cause of preventable death in the United States. Worldwide, tobacco use causes more than 7 million deaths each year, and it is responsible for more than 480,000 deaths annually in the United States, including more than 41,000 deaths resulting from exposure to secondhand smoke (HHS, 2014; World Health Organization, 2017). In addition, more than 16 million Americans are living with a disease caused by smoking (HHS, 2014). On average, smokers die at least 10 years earlier than nonsmokers (Jha et al., 2013), and according to the U.S. Surgeon General, if smoking continues at the current rate among U.S. youth, 5.6 million of today's Americans under age 18 are expected to die prematurely from a smoking-related illness (HHS, 2014).

Tobacco use among adolescents is related to a number of negative health outcomes. Youth smoking is strongly associated with depression, anxiety, and stress, such that smoking may precede or develop as a result of these mental and emotional health problems. Youth smoking can also lead to increased respiratory illnesses, decreased physical fitness, and detrimental effects on lung growth and function (HHS, 2012). If continued into adulthood, smoking can lead to disease and disability in nearly every organ of the body. Indeed, the major causes of excess mortality among smokers are diseases that are related to smoking, including cancer, respiratory disease, and vascular disease (HHS, 2014).

Use of tobacco products typically begins during adolescence, with nearly 9 of 10 cigarette smokers trying their first cigarette by age 18 (HHS, 2014). Fortunately, combustible cigarette use among youth has been decreasing over the last 20 years. The YRBSS has documented a significant decrease in the prevalence of having ever tried a cigarette between 1991 (70.1%) and 2017 (28.9%; Kann et al., 2018) (see Figure 3-5).

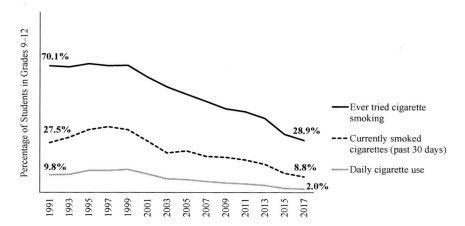

FIGURE 3-5 Cigarette use among high schoolers has decreased significantly since 1999.
NOTES: The Youth Risk Behavior Survey asked about cigarette use before age 13 only in 2017 (9.5%; Kann et al., 2018). See Figure 3-6 below for data from the National Youth Tobacco Survey on trends in cigarette use for middle school students.
SOURCE: Generated using Youth Risk Behavior Survey data (CDC, 2019b).

However, overall tobacco use has been increasing. According to the NYTS, 7.2 percent of middle school students and 27.1 percent of high school students reported current use of any tobacco product (past 30 days) in 2018, compared with 6.5 percent of middle school students and 22.9 percent of high school students in 2013 (Arrazola et al., 2014; Gentzke et al., 2019).[7]

This increase in adolescent tobacco use is most notably related to electronic vapor products, including e-cigarettes, e-cigars, e-pipes, vape pipes, vaping pens, e-hookahs, and hookah pens. E-cigarettes entered the U.S. marketplace in 2006 as an alternative to cigarettes (Cahn and Siegel, 2011; HHS, 2016a). By 2014, e-cigarettes were the most commonly used tobacco product among U.S. youth, and their use in this population has continued to increase (HHS, 2016a). In 2018, 20.8 percent of high school and 4.9 percent of middle school students reported current e-cigarette use, compared with 1.5 percent and 0.6 percent, respectively, in 2011 (Gentzke et al., 2019) (see Figure 3-6). Given concerns about health, nicotine exposure, nicotine dependence, and the transition to combustible tobacco products,

---

[7]Trends in current tobacco and e-cigarette use are from the NYTS because this survey provides the most up-to-date information on the rapidly growing e-cigarette epidemic.

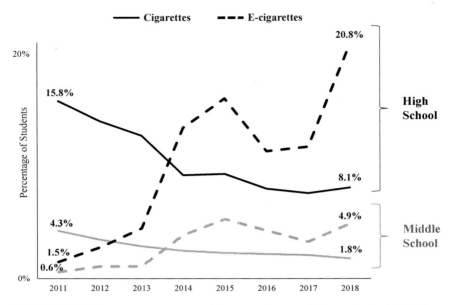

FIGURE 3-6 E-cigarette use among adolescents increased dramatically in 2018.
SOURCE: Generated using National Youth Tobacco Survey data, as presented by
Gentzke et al. (2019), Jamal et al. (2017), and HHS (2016a).

the U.S. Surgeon General and the Food and Drug Administration (FDA)
commissioner have declared e-cigarette use among youth to be a public
health epidemic (HHS, 2018b; U.S. Food and Drug Administration, 2018a).
   Current e-cigarette use varies by biological sex and race/ethnicity. In
2018, current use was higher for males in both high school (22.6%) and
middle school (5.1%) compared with their female peers (18.8% and 4.9%,
respectively). With respect to race/ethnicity, more white high schoolers
reported current e-cigarette use (26.8%) compared with their black (7.5%)
and Hispanic (14.8%) counterparts. However, current e-cigarette use among
middle schoolers was highest among Hispanic (6.6%) compared with white
(4.9%) and black (3.0%) students (Gentzke et al., 2019) (see Figure 3-7).
   Adolescent perceptions of the health risks associated with e-cigarettes
can affect their use. In general, research shows that the main factors
accounting for why adolescents are more susceptible than other groups to
initiating use of tobacco products are flavors; marketing; social pressures;
and the belief that alternative tobacco products, such as e-cigarettes, are not
harmful (Ambrose et al., 2014; Amrock, Lee, and Weitzman, 2016; Cooper
et al., 2016; Gorukanti et al., 2017; Harrell et al., 2017; Hebert et al.,

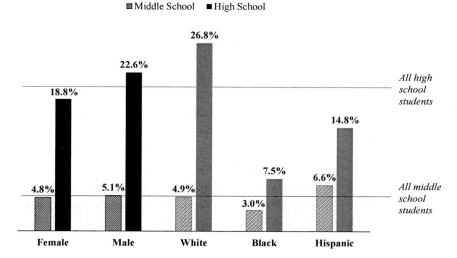

FIGURE 3-7 E-cigarette use in the past 30 days was highest among males and lowest among black adolescents in 2018.
NOTES: Data for other specific racial/ethnic populations were not available in this source.
"Other race" was excluded because (1) middle school data are not available, and (2) the significant heterogeneity of this group limits the conclusions that can be drawn.
SOURCE: Generated using National Youth Tobacco Survey data, as presented by Gentzke et al. (2019).

2017; McKelvey, Baiocchi, and Halpern-Felsher, 2018; Meyers, Delucchi, and Halpern-Felsher, 2017; Nguyen, McKelvey, and Halpern-Felsher, 2019; Pepper, Ribisl, and Brewer, 2016; Roditis et al., 2016; Schaefer, Adams, and Haas, 2013). Among modern e-cigarette devices, the most well-known is JUUL, which was first introduced in 2015 and has quickly become the most common device used by youth because of its sleek design, user-friendly function, desirable flavors, and ability to be used discreetly (Fadus, Smith, and Squeglia, 2019; Kavuluru, Han, and Hahn, 2019; Willett et al., 2019).

As opposed to many adult smokers, a large percentage of youth who have used e-cigarettes have never tried traditional cigarettes (Hughes et al., 2015). Additionally, e-cigarettes drive many adolescents to become dual or poly tobacco product users. Among adolescent e-cigarette users, 75 percent reported concurrent use of other forms of tobacco (Anand et al., 2015). This is important because youth who use multiple tobacco products have been found to be at higher risk for developing nicotine dependence and continuing tobacco use into adulthood (HHS, 2012).

E-cigarette vapor contains many of the same harmful toxins as traditional cigarettes (NASEM, 2018b). However, the safety and long-term effects of e-cigarettes are still vague. The CDC and FDA, along with state and local health departments and other partners from the health sector, are currently responding to a national outbreak of e-cigarette or vaping product use–associated lung injuries (EVALI). Current evidence suggests that EVALI may be associated with THC-containing products. This outbreak aside, however, the CDC reiterates that e-cigarette or vaping products should never be used by youth (CDC, 2019e).

Social and Environmental Influences

Risk factors associated with cigarette use include risk perceptions, social influences from family and friends, and individual affective characteristics such as depression and sensation seeking (Wellman et al., 2016). A recent study found that the most common trends in characteristics of adolescent e-cigarette users are being male, older age, having more pocket money, and having peers who smoke (Perikleous et al., 2018).

Parental influences are strongly related to adolescent tobacco use. Young people may be more likely to use tobacco products if one of their parents uses cigarettes or smokeless tobacco products (Vassoler and Sadri-Vakili, 2014). Lack of support or involvement from parents is also associated with youth tobacco use (HHS, 2012, 2016a).

Adolescents are more also likely to use tobacco products if they see peers using these products and are more motivated to participate in social smoking compared with adult smokers (Bonilha et al., 2013). There is also concern that e-cigarette use may renormalize a smoking culture among young people, subverting decades of antismoking efforts (Bell and Keane, 2014; Kandel and Kandel, 2015; Stanwick, 2015).

Just as the media play an enormous role in underage drinking, they portray tobacco use as normative. Manufacturers and retailers of tobacco products market aggressively to youth through the Internet, social media, television, radio, event sponsorship, celebrity placement, and strategic positioning in convenience stores (Cobb, Brookover, and Cobb, 2015; de Andrade, Hastings, and Angus, 2013; Grana and Ling, 2014). In particular, much of the rise in the popularity of e-cigarettes has stemmed from innovative advertising campaigns that target adolescents through social media (Jackler et al., 2019; Mantey et al., 2016). An analysis of e-cigarette retail websites and marketing and promotional campaigns revealed recurrent appeals to adolescents, such as use by celebrities, feature cartoons, and sexual appeal (Grana and Ling, 2014).

The active enforcement of youth access laws is critical to preventing adolescent tobacco use. E-cigarettes are illegal to purchase under the age of 18, and even 21 in many states (Morain and Malek, 2017; Murthy, 2017; Wang et al., 2014). However, youth frequently report purchasing these devices from retail locations in person as well as online (Mantey et al., 2019; Meyers, Delucchi, and Halpern-Felsher, 2017). As of November 2018, a new FDA regulation requires stronger age verification for online sales of e-cigarettes, as well as the removal of e-cigarette products from the market that are marketed to children or are appealing to youth (U.S. Food and Drug Administration, 2018b).

Sexual Behavior in Adolescence

Trends

First sexual intercourse, or sexual debut, is an important milestone in sexual and human development. While there appear to be no consistent negative consequences of protected and consensual intercourse between adolescents, the empirical literature reflects broad consensus that earlier age of first intercourse is associated with a higher risk of not using contraception, not using barrier methods of protection against STIs, and higher rates of unintended pregnancy and STIs (Burke, Gabhainn, and Kelly, 2018; Santelli et al., 2017).

The prevalence of sexual intercourse among adolescents has decreased overall since 1991 (CDC, 2019b) (see Figure 3-8).[8] According to the YRBS, the percentage of students in grades 9–12 who reported ever having sexual intercourse decreased from 54.1 percent in 1991 to 39.5 percent in 2017 (CDC, 2019b). In the same time period, the percentage who first had sexual intercourse before age 13 decreased from 10.2 percent to 3.4 percent. Among those reporting sexual experience, the percentage who were currently sexually active (in the past 3 months) also decreased overall, from 37.5 percent to 28.7 percent, and the percentage who had had sexual intercourse with four or more people in their lifetime decreased from 18.7 percent to 9.7 percent. These decreasing trends were consistent by both biological sex and race/ethnicity.

Research has shown that those who engage in vaginal sex at an earlier age also have more sexual partners (Sandfort et al., 2008). However, more recent research also suggests that numbers of sexual partners may be more consequential for health outcomes than age at sexual debut. Kahn and Halpern (2018) found that those who initiated sex early but had fewer lifetime partners exhibited better health outcomes from adolescence to early adulthood, including fewer STI/sexually transmitted disease (STD) diagnoses

---

[8]As noted previously, "sexual intercourse" is not defined in the YRBS. The result can be biased estimates, particularly for LGBTQ youth.

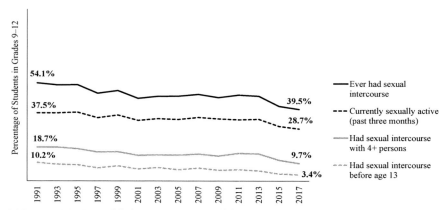

FIGURE 3-8 Sexual behaviors among adolescents decreased from 1991 to 2017.
SOURCE: Generated using Youth Risk Behavior Survey data (CDC, 2019b).

and unintended pregnancies and better romantic relationship quality relative to those who initiated later but reported more sexual partners.

With respect to sexuality in relation to adolescent risk taking, risk factors associated with sexual activity among adolescents are those that increase the likelihood of unintended pregnancy and/or an STI. Teenagers can reduce their chances of experiencing these outcomes by using proper and effective contraception. Indeed, cross-national research suggests that most teenagers can engage safely in sexual behavior if provided with adequate access to contraception and sexual education (Harden, 2014; Santelli, Sandfort, and Orr, 2008). Unfortunately, the potential negative or unintended consequences of unprotected sexual behavior, such as having an unintended pregnancy or acquiring an STI, affect adolescents disproportionately (NASEM, 2019).

In every YRBS year, a consistent majority of sexually active adolescents reported using a method to prevent pregnancy, whether condoms or some other method, at last sexual intercourse. Furthermore, use of any method increased overall from 1991 (83.5%) to 2017 (86.2%). However, despite greater increases in use of contraception among black/African American (76.0% to 82.2%) and Hispanic (74.4% to 81.0%) adolescents compared with their white counterparts (87.4% to 90.0%), overall disparities still exist among these racial/ethnic groups (CDC, 2019b) (see Figure 3-9).[9]

Although YRBS data suggest a number of promising trends in sexual behavior among adolescents, including later onset of sexual intercourse, fewer lifetime sexual partners, and high rates of contraceptive use

---

[9]There were insufficient data to report trends for American Indian/Alaska Native, Asian, and Native Hawaiian/Pacific Islander populations.

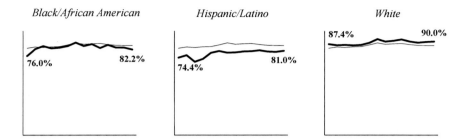

FIGURE 3-9 Despite increases in the use of any method to prevent pregnancy among sexually active adolescents from 1991 to 2017, overall racial/ethnic disparities persist.
NOTE: Consistent data for American Indian/Alaska Native, Asian, and Native Hawaiian/Pacific Islander populations were not available for this Youth Risk Behavior Survey item.
SOURCE: Generated using Youth Risk Behavior Survey data (CDC, 2019b).

among both males and females and across racial/ethnic groups, condom use among sexually active adolescents fell from 61.5 percent in 2007 to 53.8 percent in 2017 (CDC, 2019b). Importantly, while the proportion of sexually active adolescents who used effective hormonal birth control (long-acting reversible contraceptives [LARCs] or other hormonal methods) increased by 4.1 percent from 2013 to 2017 (CDC, 2019b), these forms of contraception are not effective against STIs. Dual protection (a condom and a hormonal birth control method) can help prevent both STIs and pregnancy; consistently, however, only 8.8 percent of sexually active high school students reported using both a condom and effective hormonal birth control at last intercourse (Kann et al., 2018) (see Figure 3-10).

Health Outcomes Associated with Sexual Behavior During Adolescence

As noted, both unintended pregnancy and STIs/STDs are among the most important adverse health outcomes associated with sexual behavior.

Pregnancy

Pregnancy and birth rates among 15- to 19-year-olds in the United States have decreased over time (CDC, 2018d; Kost, Maddow-Zimet, and Arpaia, 2017; Martin et al., 2018). Between 1991 and 2013, pregnancy rates for all 15- to 19-year-old females decreased from 115.9 to 43.4 per 1,000, while pregnancy rates among sexually experienced females decreased from 223.1 to 101.2 per 1,000. Birth rates also decreased, from 61.8 per

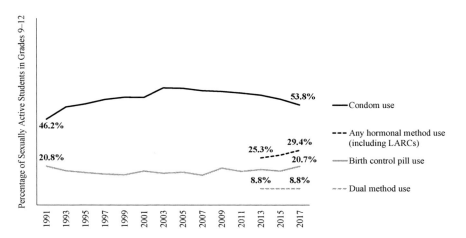

FIGURE 3-10 Use of hormonal birth control has increased, but dual-method use (condom and hormonal method) has remained unchanged.
SOURCE: Generated using Youth Risk Behavior Survey data (CDC, 2019b).

1,000 in 1991 to 18.8 per 1,000 in 2017 (CDC, 2018d; Martin et al., 2018) (see Figure 3-11).

Much of the decrease in the teen pregnancy and birth rates has been attributed to greater access to contraception rather than to overall reductions in sexual behavior (Lindberg, Santelli, and Desai, 2016, 2018; Santelli et al., 2007). Furthermore, recent research suggests that reality television, such as the MTV shows "16 and Pregnant" and "Teen Mom," which depict the struggles of teen mothers, may have contributed to up to a third of the decline in teenage births between when they first aired in 2009 and 2010 (Kearney and Levine, 2015).

Despite promising trends overall, racial and ethnic differences in teen pregnancy and birth rates persist. In 2013, teen pregnancy rates were 76.1 per 1,000 for black adolescents and 60.8 per 1,000 for Hispanic adolescents, compared with 37.6 per 1,000 for white adolescents (Kost, Maddow-Zimet, and Arpaia, 2017) (see Figure 3-12). In 2017, birth rates were 27.5 per 1,000 for black adolescents and 28.9 per 1,000 for Hispanic adolescents, compared with 13.2 per 1,000 for white adolescents (CDC, 2018d; Martin et al., 2018) (refer to Figure 3-12). Although much progress has been made in reducing teen pregnancy overall, these significant racial/ethnic disparities indicate that black/African American and Hispanic/Latino female adolescents still need additional services and supports.

Social and economic disadvantage are strongly associated with disparities in teen pregnancy and birth rates (Kearney and Levine, 2012). For

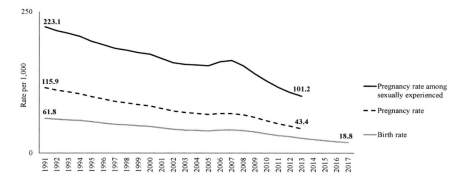

FIGURE 3-11 Teen pregnancy and birth rates decreased from 1991 to 2013.
SOURCE: Generated using pregnancy data from the National Survey of Family Growth, as analyzed by Kost, Maddow-Zimet, and Arpaia (2017) and birth surveillance data from the Centers for Disease Control and Prevention (2018d) and Martin et al. (2018).

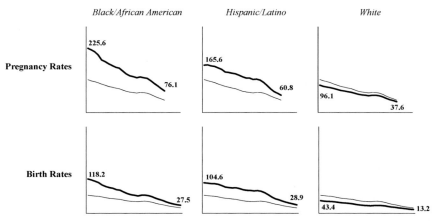

FIGURE 3-12 Despite significant decreases in pregnancy from 1991 to 2013 and birth rates from 1991 to 2017 among 15- to 19-year-olds, racial/ethnic disparities persist.
NOTES: Pregnancy rate data for other racial/ethnic populations were not available in this source.

"Other" race was excluded because (1) the composition of this group varies by data source, and (2) the significant heterogeneity of this group limits the conclusions that can be drawn.
SOURCES: Generated using pregnancy data from the National Survey of Family Growth, as analyzed by Kost, Maddow-Zimet, and Arpaia (2017) and birth surveillance data from the Centers for Disease Control and Prevention (2018d) and Martin et al. (2018).

example, adolescents who are in child welfare systems are at a higher risk of teenage pregnancy and birth relative to other groups (Boonstra, 2011). Additionally, adolescents living in lower-income neighborhoods with high levels of unemployment are more likely to become pregnant and give birth compared with adolescents living in neighborhoods with greater income and employment opportunities (Penman-Aguilar et al., 2013).

A variety of evidence-based teen pregnancy prevention programs and interventions, including a number of those on the TPP registry of programs, have shown effectiveness in preventing unintended teen pregnancies in diverse populations and settings (Fish et al., 2014; Lugo-Gil et al., 2018). In addition to prevention programs, adolescents need support from parents and other trusted adults in making healthy choices about relationships, sex, and birth control. Adolescents also need access to youth-friendly contraceptive and reproductive health services. Community efforts to address the social and economic factors associated with teenage pregnancy can play a major role as well in tackling racial/ethnic and geographic disparities in teen birth rates (CDC, 2019f; Kearney and Levine, 2012).

Sexually Transmitted Infections and Diseases

The United States has the highest rate of STIs in the industrialized world. A combination of behavioral, biological, and cultural factors put sexually active adolescents at higher risk of contracting STIs compared with other age groups. Young people ages 15 to 24 account for nearly half of all new cases of STIs each year (CDC, 2018e). In particular, female and black young people are significantly more likely to contract an STI (CDC, 2018e, 2018f).

The most effective way to prevent STIs is to abstain from sexual activity. For those who are sexually active, using a condom correctly every time one has sex can reduce the likelihood of contracting an STI. Yet while condoms are the most effective way to prevent STIs, they are not the most effective way to prevent pregnancy. As mentioned previously, the best way to prevent both STIs and pregnancy is using dual protection, defined as using both a condom and a form of hormonal birth control (CDC, 2018g).

The most common STIs among young people in the United States are chlamydia and gonorrhea. Chlamydia rates among 15- to 19-year-olds have increased over time, from 1,126.3 per 100,000 in 1997 to 2,110.6 per 100,000 in 2018, peaking at 2,082.7 per 100,000 in 2011. In contrast, gonorrhea rates per 100,000 15- to 19-year-olds decreased from 1997 (530.3) to 2014 (325.0), but increased from 2014 to 2017 (438.2) (CDC, 2019g, 2019h) (see Figure 3-13).

There are also significant and persistent disparities in chlamydia and gonorrhea rates among 15- to 19-year-olds by race/ethnicity, with sig-

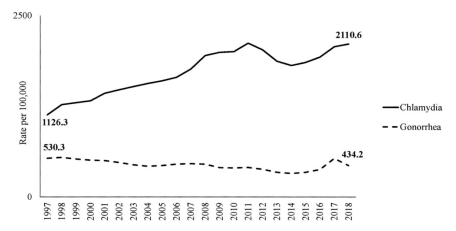

FIGURE 3-13 Chlamydia rates among 15- to 19-year-olds have risen substantially since 1997, while gonorrhea rates have risen more recently.
SOURCE: Generated using sexually transmitted disease surveillance data from the Centers for Disease Control and Prevention (2019g, 2019h).

nificantly higher rates among black teens at every time point. In 2018, chlamydia rates per 100,000 for black youth were 4,714.8, compared with 2,445.7 for American Indian/Alaska Native, 327.9 for Asian, 1,134.9 for Hispanic/Latino, and 890.7 for white adolescents. Similarly, gonorrhea rates per 100,000 were highest among black adolescents (1,457.7), followed by American Indian/Alaska Native (554.9), Hispanic/Latino (188.6), white (132.9) and Asian (47.8) youth (CDC, 2019g, 2019h) (see Figure 3-14).

Social and Environmental Influences

As mentioned in Chapter 1, sexual development is distinctly different from alcohol and tobacco use because it represents a critical task of adolescence. As a part of their sexual development, adolescents typically form intimate partnerships, affirm gender identities, identify sexual orientations, situate sexuality in the context of their religious beliefs, and incorporate cultural attitudes toward sexuality into their own value systems, all of which help them prepare for adult roles and relationships (Diamond and Savin-Williams, 2009; Everett, 2019; NASEM, 2019; Suleiman et al, 2017; Tulloch and Kaufman, 2013).

Based on growing scientific evidence, sexual activity is increasingly considered a normative aspect of adolescent development (NASEM, 2019; Tolman and McClelland, 2011). However, rather than navigating a binary

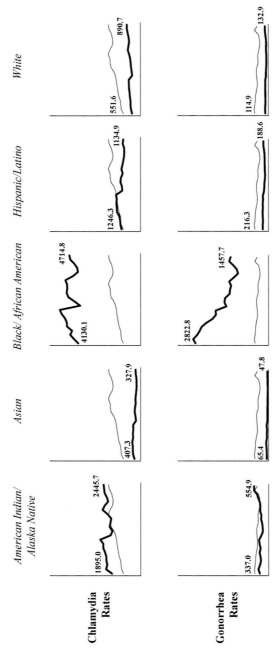

FIGURE 3-14 Chlamydia and gonorrhea rates per 100,000 15- to 19-year-olds are significantly and consistently higher among black/African American youth compared with their counterparts from other racial/ethnic groups (1997 to 2018).
SOURCE: Generated using sexually transmitted disease surveillance data from the Centers for Disease Control and Prevention (2019g, 2019h).

division between positive or risky, adolescent sexual activity can be characterized as both positive and risky. This framework embraces the reality that adolescents must learn about themselves, their bodies, intimate partners, and relationships within contexts in which they are required to both manage risks and develop positive patterns for sexuality into adulthood (Harden, 2014; Tolman and McClelland, 2011).

While unhealthy risk behaviors can occur within a sexual context, having sex is not necessarily unhealthy or problematic, even in adolescence. However, this does not imply that all sexual activity is healthy and positive or that abstinence is unhealthy. Rather, whether sexual behaviors are labeled "healthy" or "unhealthy" is highly dependent on the individual, the context, and cultural influences (Harden, 2014; Tolman and McClelland, 2011).

Parental attitudes toward sexuality and parenting style are important factors contributing to an adolescent's sexual attitudes and behaviors, as parents typically serve as models for normative behaviors and attitudes (Tulloch and Kaufman, 2013). Parents can also support healthy sexual development by providing age- and developmentally appropriate information on sexual topics including puberty, reproduction, pregnancy prevention, STIs, healthy relationships, sexual orientation, gender identity, consent, boundaries, and body image. Furthermore, parents can help adolescents build critical thinking skills with which to assess the reliability of sexual information portrayed in the media, teach them about their rights and responsibilities in romantic relationships and sexual activities, and address ways to deal with peer pressure (Ashcraft and Murray, 2017; Berkel, 2019; Hagan, Shaw, and Duncan, 2017; McNeely and Blanchard, 2010; NASEM, 2019).

Adolescents also use peers as a resource to learn about sexuality (McNeely and Blanchard, 2010; Tolman and McClelland, 2011). Unfortunately, peers can be a source of inaccurate and misleading information. For instance, many adolescents overestimate the sexual activity of their peers, which can result in feeling pressured to "catch up" (Warner et al., 2011). Peers often exert pressure to conform to the "normal behavior" of their peer group. An adolescent's sexual activities or experience can also affect social standing, leading to damaging rumors, peer group rejection, partner rejection, regret or remorse, vulnerability, and depression.

Physicians can also play a role in an adolescent's understanding of sexuality. According to the CDC (2018h), six major elements are involved in youth-friendly sexual and reproductive health services: (1) confidentiality, (2) privacy, (3) consent, (4) cultural and linguistic appropriateness, (5) comprehensive services, and (6) parent/guardian involvement. The best services provide youth with clear, accurate information about their rights, make them feel respected and engaged in their health care, and address their contraceptive and reproductive health needs at every visit (CDC, 2018h). Adolescents with developmental disabilities, chronic health conditions, or physical disabilities in particular may benefit from these services, as conversations with physicians may be one of the only ways they can receive accurate information related to sexuality and their conditions (Horner-Johnson and Sauvé, 2019).

Finally, the prominent and multifaceted role of the media in adolescent sexual development is one of the greatest differences between today's adolescents and those of prior generations. Adolescents can access a large amount of sexual content online, some of which is misleading and can lead to unhealthy sexual behaviors. In recent decades, moreover, adolescents have had more access to literature related to sexuality, to media coverage of sexual crimes and violence, and to portrayals of sexuality on television and the Internet (Harris, 2011). Media use can also facilitate dating and romantic relationships. In particular, dating apps and websites have revolutionized how people meet and engage, and access to technology and social media has made it even easier to establish and maintain romantic relationships (Lenhart and Duggan, 2014; Seemiller and Grace, 2018).

CONCLUSIONS

Based on the findings presented in this chapter, the committee drew the following conclusions.

CONCLUSION 3-1: Risk-taking activities are a normal and necessary part of adolescence because of the heightened neurological plasticity of the brain that makes it especially malleable and responsive to experiences, as well as the developmental purpose of such activities of preparing youth for adulthood. Therefore, "discontinuation of risk" is applicable only to those unhealthy risk behaviors (e.g., substance abuse, unprotected sexual activity) that can lead to negative health outcomes (e.g., diseases, unintended pregnancy, sexually transmitted infections).

CONCLUSION 3-2: The current Youth Risk Behavior Survey does not reflect the experiences of out-of-school adolescents (e.g., dropped out, homeless), many of whom are more likely to engage or have engaged in unhealthy risk behaviors.

CONCLUSION 3-3: The sexual behavior items included in the Youth Risk Behavior Survey are neither specific nor comprehensive enough to (1) provide the most accurate estimates of the sexual behaviors in which today's youth engage and (2) represent the experiences of LGBTQ populations.

CONCLUSION 3-4: There are significant racial and ethnic disparities in health behaviors and outcomes, which are related to differences in access to opportunities and supports (see Conclusion 2-1 in Chapter 2). Therefore, disadvantaged youth need more resources to reduce such disparities and ensure access to comparable opportunities (see Conclusion 2-3 in Chapter 2).

CONCLUSION 3-5: Unlike alcohol and tobacco use, sexual development represents a critical developmental task that prepares adolescents for adult roles and relationships. It is therefore just as important to support healthy sexual development as it is to prevent the negative health outcomes associated with sexual behavior (e.g., unintended pregnancy, sexually transmitted infections) during adolescence.

The next chapter of this report documents the process and findings of the committee's review of core components of programs and interventions that have been found to be successful in promoting positive health behaviors and outcomes among adolescents using the optimal health framework.

REFERENCES

Adger Jr., H., and Saha, S. (2013). Alcohol use disorders in adolescents. *Pediatrics in Review, 34*(3), 103–113.

Albert, D., Chein, J., and Steinberg, L. (2013). The teenage brain: Peer influences on adolescent decision making. *Current Directions in Psychological Science, 22*(2), 114–120.

Ambrose, B.K., Rostron, B.L., Johnson, S.E., Portnoy, D.B., Apelberg, B.J., Kaufman, A.R., and Choiniere, C.J. (2014). Perceptions of the relative harm of cigarettes and e-cigarettes among U.S. youth. *American Journal of Preventive Medicine, 47*(2 Suppl 1), S53–S60.

Amrock, S.M., Lee, L., and Weitzman, M. (2016). Perceptions of e-cigarettes and noncigarette tobacco products among U.S. youth. *Pediatrics, 138*(5).

Anand, V., McGinty, K.L., O'Brien, K., Guenthner, G., Hahn, E., and Martin, C.A. (2015). E-cigarette use and beliefs among urban public high school students in North Carolina. *Journal of Adolescent Health, 57*(1), 46–51.

Arrazola, R.A., Neff, L.J., Kennedy, S.M., Holder-Hayes, E., and Jones, C.D. (2014). Tobacco use among middle and high school students—United States, 2013. *Morbidity and Mortality Weekly Report, 63*(45), 1021–1026.

Ashcraft, A.M., and Murray, P.J. (2017). Talking to parents about adolescent sexuality. *Pediatric Clinics of North America, 64*(2), 305–320.

Bell, K., and Keane, H. (2014). All gates lead to smoking: The 'gateway theory,' e-cigarettes and the remaking of nicotine. *Social Science & Medicine, 119*, 45–52.

Berkel, C. (2019). *The Role of Sexual Agency and Consent in Healthy Adolescent Development.* Paper commissioned by the Committee on Applying Lessons of Optimal Adolescent Health to Improve Behavioral Outcomes for Youth. Available: https://www.nap.edu/resource/25552/The%20Role%20of%20Sexual%20Agency%20and%20Consent%20in%20Healthy%20Adolescent%20Development.pdf.

Blakemore, S-J. (2018). Avoiding social risk in adolescence. *Current Directions in Psychological Science, 27*(2), 116–122.

Blakemore, S-J., and Robbins, T.W. (2012). Decision-making in the adolescent brain. *Nature Neuroscience, 15*, 1184.

Bonilha, A.G., de Souza, E.S., Sicchieri, M.P., Achcar, J.A., Crippa, J.A., and Baddini-Martinez, J. (2013). A motivational profile for smoking among adolescents. *Journal of Addiction Medicine, 7*(6), 439–446.

Boonstra, H.D. (2011). Teen pregnancy among young women in foster care: A primer. *Policy Review, 14*(2), 8–19.

Braams, B.R., van Duijvenvoorde, A.C., Peper, J.S., and Crone, E.A. (2015). Longitudinal changes in adolescent risk-taking: A comprehensive study of neural responses to rewards, pubertal development, and risk-taking behavior. *Journal of Neuroscience, 35*(18), 7226–7238.

Brener, N.D., Eaton, D.K., Kann, L., Grunbaum, J.A., Gross, L.A., Kyle, T.M., and Ross, J.G. (2006). The association of survey setting and mode with self-reported health risk behaviors among high school students. *Public Opinion Quarterly, 70*(3), 354–374.

Brener, N.D., Kann, L., Shanklin, S., Kinchen, S., Eaton, D.K., Hawkins, J., and Flint, K.H. (2013). Methodology of the Youth Risk Behavior Surveillance System—2013. *Morbidity and Mortality Weekly Report: Recommendations and Reports, 62*(1), 1–20.

Bronfenbrenner, U. (1994). Ecological models of human development. *Readings on the Development of Children, 2*(1), 37–43.

Burke, L., Gabhainn, S.N., and Kelly, C. (2018). Socio-demographic, health and lifestyle factors influencing age of sexual initiation among adolescents. *International Journal of Environmental Research and Public Health, 15*(9).

Cahn, Z. and Siegel, M. (2011). Electronic cigarettes as a harm reduction strategy for tobacco control: A step forward or a repeat of past mistakes? *Journal of Public Health Policy, 32*(1), 16–31.

Catalano, R.F., Fagan, A.A., Gavin, L.E., Greenberg, M.T., Irwin Jr., C.E., Ross, D.A., and Shek, D.T.L. (2012). Worldwide application of prevention science in adolescent health. *The Lancet, 379*(9826), 1653–1664.

Centers for Disease Control and Prevention (CDC). (2018a). *School Connectedness.* Available: https://www.cdc.gov/healthyyouth/protective/school_connectedness.htm.

———. (2018b). *Youth Risk Behavior Surveillance System (YRBSS) Overview.* Available: https://www.cdc.gov/healthyyouth/data/yrbs/overview.htm.

———. (2018c). *YRBS Questionnaires: 1991–2019.* Atlanta, GA: Author.

———. (2018d). *Birth Rates for Females by Age Group: United States.* Hyattsville, MD: Author.

———. (2018e). STDs in adolescents and young adults. *Sexually Transmitted Disease Surveillance 2017: Special Focus Profiles.* Available: https://www.cdc.gov/std/stats17/adolescents.htm.

———. (2018f). STDs in racial and ethnic minorities. *Sexually Transmitted Disease Surveillance 2017: Special Focus Profiles* Available: https://www.cdc.gov/std/stats17/minorities.htm.

———. (2018g). *Contraception.* Available: https://www.cdc.gov/reproductivehealth/contraception/index.htm.

———. (2018h). *Teen-Friendly Reproductive Health Visit.* Available: https://www.cdc.gov/teenpregnancy/health-care-providers/teen-friendly-health-visit.htm.

———. (2019a). *Youth Violence.* Available: https://www.cdc.gov/violenceprevention/youthviolence/index.html.

———. (2019b). *Youth Risk Behavior Surveillance System (YRBSS) Youth Online High School Results.* Available: https://nccd.cdc.gov/Youthonline/App/Results.aspx.

———. (2019c). *Leading Causes of Death Reports, 1981–2017.* Available: https://webappa.cdc.gov/sasweb/ncipc/leadcause.html.

———. (2019d). *Teen Drivers: Get the Facts.* Available: https://www.cdc.gov/motorvehiclesafety/teen_drivers/teendrivers_factsheet.html.

———. (2019e). *Outbreak of Lung Injury Associated with the Use of E-cigarette, or Vaping, Products.* Available: https://www.cdc.gov/tobacco/basic_information/e-cigarettes/severe-lung-disease.html.

———. (2019f). *Social Determinants and Eliminating Disparities in Teen Pregnancy.* Available: https://www.cdc.gov/teenpregnancy/about/social-determinants-disparities-teen-pregnancy.htm.

———. (2019g). *CDC Sexually Transmitted Diseases (STDs) Data and Statistics–Archive.* Available: https://www.cdc.gov/std/stats/archive.htm.

———. (2019h). *Sexually Transmitted Disease Surveillance 2018.* Atlanta, GA: Author.

Chung, T., Creswell, K.G., Bachrach, R., Clark, D.B., and Martin, C.S. (2018). Adolescent binge drinking. *Alcohol Research, 39*(1), 5–15.

Cobb, N.K., Brookover, J., and Cobb, C.O. (2015). Forensic analysis of online marketing for electronic nicotine delivery systems. *Tobacco Control, 24*(2), 128–131.

Cooper, M., Harrell, M.B., Perez, A., Delk, J., and Perry, C.L. (2016). Flavorings and perceived harm and addictiveness of e-cigarettes among youth. *Tobacco Regulatory Science, 2*(3), 278–289.

Cross, S.J., Lotfipour, S., and Leslie, F.M. (2017). Mechanisms and genetic factors underlying co-use of nicotine and alcohol or other drugs of abuse. *American Journal of Drug and Alcohol Abuse, 43*(2), 171–185.

Curtin, S.C., Heron, M., Minino, A.M., and Warner, M. (2018). Recent increases in injury mortality among children and adolescents aged 10–19 years in the United States: 1999–2016. *National Vital Statistics Reports, 67*(4), 1–16.

David-Ferdon, C., Vivolo-Kantor, A.M., Dahlberg, L.L., Marshall, K.J., Rainford, N., and Hall, J.E. (2016). *A Comprehensive Technical Package for the Prevention of Youth Violence and Associated Risk Behaviors.* Atlanta, GA: U.S. Department of Health and Human Services, Centers for Disease Control and Prevention.

de Andrade, M., Hastings, G., and Angus, K. (2013). Promotion of electronic cigarettes: Tobacco marketing reinvented? *British Medical Journal, 347*, f7473.

Denniston, M.M., Brener, N.D., Kann, L., Eaton, D.K., McManus, T., Kyle, T.M., Roberts, A.M., Flint, K.H., and Ross, J.G. (2010). Comparison of paper-and-pencil versus web administration of the Youth Risk Behavior Survey (YRBS): Participation, data quality, and perceived privacy and anonymity. *Computers in Human Behavior, 26*(5), 1054–1060.

Diamond, L.M., and Savin-Williams, R.C. (2009). Adolescent sexuality. In R.M. Lerner and L. Steinberg (Eds.), *Handbook of Adolescent Psychology: Individual Bases of Adolescent Development* (pp. 479–524). Hoboken, NJ: John Wiley & Sons, Inc.

Duell, N., and Steinberg, L. (2019). Positive risk taking in adolescence. *Child Development Perspectives, 13*(1), 48–52.

Eaton, D.K., Brener, N.D., Kann, L., Denniston, M.M., McManus, T., Kyle, T.M., Roberts, A.M., Flint, K.H., and Ross, J.G. (2010). Comparison of paper-and-pencil versus web administration of the Youth Risk Behavior Survey (YRBS): Risk behavior prevalence estimates. *Evaluation Review, 34*(2), 137–153.

Edidin, J.P., Ganim, Z., Hunter, S.J., and Karnik, N.S. (2012). The mental and physical health of homeless youth: A literature review. *Child Psychiatry & Human Development, 43*(3), 354–375.

Everett, B.G. (2019). *Optimal Adolescent Health to Improve Behavioral Outcomes for LGBTQ Youth.* Paper commissioned by the Committee on Applying Lessons of Optimal Adolescent Health to Improve Behavioral Outcomes for Youth. Available: https://www.nap.edu/resource/25552/Optimal%20Adolescent%20Health%20to%20Improve%20Behavioral%20Outcomes%20for%20LGBTQ%20Youth.pdf.

Fadus, M.C., Smith, T.T., and Squeglia, L.M. (2019). The rise of e-cigarettes, pod mod devices, and JUUL among youth: Factors influencing use, health implications, and downstream effects. *Drug and Alcohol Dependence, 201*, 85–93.

Falk, E.B., Cascio, C.N., O'Donnell, M.B., Carp, J., Tinney Jr., F.J., Bingham, C.R., Shope, J.T., Ouimet, M.C., Pradhan, A.K., and Simons-Morton, B.G. (2014). Neural responses to exclusion predict susceptibility to social influence. *Journal of Adolescent Health, 54*(5 Suppl), S22–S31.

Fish, H., Manlove, J., Moore, K.A., and Mass, E. (2014). *What Works for Adolescent Sexual and Reproductive Health: Lessons from Experimental Evaluations of Programs and Interventions.* Bethesda, MD: Child Trends.

Fosco, G.M., Frank, J.L., Stormshak, E.A., and Dishion, T.J. (2013). Opening the "black box": Family check-up intervention effects on self-regulation that prevents growth in problem behavior and substance use. *Journal of School Psychology, 51*(4), 455–468.

Freudenberg, N. and Ruglis, J. (2007). Reframing school dropout as a public health issue. *Preventing Chronic Disease: Public Health Research, Practice, and Policy, 4*(4).

Gentzke, A.S., Creamer, M., Cullen, K.A., Ambrose, B.K., Willis, G., Jamal, A., and King, B.A. (2019). Vital signs: Tobacco product use among middle and high school students—United States, 2011–2018. *Morbidity and Mortality Weekly Report, 68*(6), 157–164.

Gershon, P., Zhu, C., Klauer, S.G., Dingus, T., and Simons-Morton, B. (2017). Teens' distracted driving behavior: Prevalence and predictors. *Journal of Safety Research, 63*, 157–161.

Gnambs, T. and Kaspar, K. (2015). Disclosure of sensitive behaviors across self-administered survey modes: A meta-analysis. *Behavior Research Methods, 47*(4), 1237–1259.

Goliath, V. and Pretorius, B. (2016). Peer risk and protective factors in adolescence: Implications for drug use prevention. *Social Work, 52*(1), 113–129.

Gorukanti, A., Delucchi, K., Ling, P., Fisher-Travis, R., and Halpern-Felsher, B. (2017). Adolescents' attitudes towards e-cigarette ingredients, safety, addictive properties, social norms, and regulation. *Preventive Medicine, 94*, 65–71.

Graber, J.A., Nichols, T.R., and Brooks-Gunn, J. (2010). Putting pubertal timing in developmental context: Implications for prevention. *Developmental Psychobiology, 52*(3), 254–262.

Grana, R.A., and Ling, P.M. (2014). "Smoking revolution": A content analysis of electronic cigarette retail websites. *American Journal of Preventive Medicine, 46*(4), 395–403.

Hagan, J.F., Shaw, J.S., and Duncan, P.M. (2017). *Bright Futures: Guidelines for Health Supervision of Infants, Children, and Adolescents* (4th ed.). Elk Grove, IL: American Academy of Pediatrics.

Harden, K.P. (2014). A sex-positive framework for research on adolescent sexuality. *Perspectives on Psychological Science, 9*(5), 455–469.

Harding, F.M., Hingson, R.W., Klitzner, M., Mosher, J.F., Brown, J., Vincent, R.M., Dahl, E., and Cannon, C.L. (2016). Underage drinking: A review of trends and prevention strategies. *American Journal of Preventive Medicine, 51*(4), S148–S157.

Harrell, M.B., Loukas, A., Jackson, C.D., Marti, C.N., and Perry, C.L. (2017). Flavored tobacco product use among youth and young adults: What if flavors didn't exist? *Tobacco Regulatory Science, 3*(2), 168–173.

Harris, A.L. (2011). Media and technology in adolescent sexual education and safety. *Journal of Obstetric, Gynecologic & Neonatal Nursing, 40*(2), 235–242.

Hartley, C.A., and Somerville, L.H. (2015). The neuroscience of adolescent decision-making. *Current Opinion in Behavioral Sciences, 5*, 108–115.

Haydon, A.A., Herring, A.H., Prinstein, M.J., and Halpern, C.T. (2012). Beyond age at first sex: Patterns of emerging sexual behavior in adolescence and young adulthood. *Journal of Adolescent Health, 50*(5), 456–463.

Hebert, E.T., Case, K.R., Kelder, S.H., Delk, J., Perry, C.L., and Harrell, M.B. (2017). Exposure and engagement with tobacco- and e-cigarette-related social media. *Journal of Adolescent Health, 61*(3), 371–377.

Heitzeg, N.A. (2009). Education or incarceration: Zero tolerance policies and the school to prison pipeline. *Forum on Public Policy, 9*(2).

Henges, A.L., and Marczinski, C.A. (2012). Impulsivity and alcohol consumption in young social drinkers. *Addictive Behaviors, 37*(2), 217–220.

Hingson, R., and White, A. (2014). New research findings since the 2007 Surgeon General's call to action to prevent and reduce underage drinking: A review. *Journal of Studies on Alcohol and Drugs, 75*(1), 158–169.

Hofmann, W., Schmeichel, B.J., and Baddeley, A.D. (2012). Executive functions and self-regulation. *Trends in Cognitive Sciences, 16*(3), 174–180.

Holmes, C., Brieant, A., Kahn, R., Deater-Deckard, K., and Kim-Spoon, J. (2019). Structural home environment effects on developmental trajectories of self-control and adolescent risk taking. *Journal of Youth and Adolescence, 48*(1), 43–55.

Horner-Johnson, W. and Sauvé, L. (2019). *Applying Lessons of Optimal Adolescent Health to Improve Behavioral Outcomes for Youth with Disabilities.* Paper commissioned by the Committee on Applying Lessons of Optimal Adolescent Health to Improve Behavioral Outcomes for Youth. Available: https://www.nap.edu/resource/25552/Applying%20Lessons%20of%20Optimal%20Adolescent%20Health%20to%20Improve%20Behavioral%20Outcomes%20for%20Youth%20with%20Disabilities.pdf.

Hughes, K., Bellis, M.A., Hardcastle, K.A., McHale, P., Bennett, A., Ireland, R., and Pike, K. (2015). Associations between e-cigarette access and smoking and drinking behaviours in teenagers. *BMC Public Health, 15*, 244.

Institute of Medicine. (2011). *The Science of Adolescent Risk-Taking: Workshop Report.* Washington, DC: The National Academies Press.

Institute of Medicine and National Research Council. (2013). *Priorities for Research to Reduce the Threat of Firearm-Related Violence.* Washington, DC: The National Academies Press.

Institute of Medicine and National Research Council. (2014). *The Evidence for Violence Prevention Across the Lifespan and Around the World: Workshop Summary.* Washington, DC: The National Academies Press.

Jackler, R.K., Li, V.Y., Cardiff, R.A.L., and Ramamurthi, D. (2019). Promotion of tobacco products on Facebook: Policy versus practice. *Tobacco Control, 28*, 67–73.

Jamal, A., Gentzke, A., Hu, S.S., Cullen, K.A., Apelberg, B.J., Homa, D.M., and King, B.A. (2017). Tobacco use among middle and high school students—United States, 2011–2016. *Morbidity and Mortality Weekly Report, 66*(23), 597–603.

Jha, P., Ramasundarahettige, C., Landsman, V., Rostron, B., Thun, M., Anderson, R.N., McAfee, T., and Peto, R. (2013). 21st-century hazards of smoking and benefits of cessation in the United States. *New England Journal of Medicine, 368*(4), 341–350.

Judd, B. (2019). *Shared Risk and Protective Factors Impacting Adolescent Behavior and Positive Development.* Anchorage, AK: Alaska Division of Behavioral Health.

Kahn, N.F., and Halpern, C.T. (2018). Associations between patterns of sexual initiation, sexual partnering, and sexual health outcomes from adolescence to early adulthood. *Archives of Sexual Behavior, 47*(6), 1791–1810.

Kandel, D., and Kandel, E. (2015). The gateway hypothesis of substance abuse: Developmental, biological and societal perspectives. *Acta Paediatrica, 104*(2), 130–137.

Kann, L., McManus, T., Harris, W.A., Shanklin, S.L., Flint, K.H., Queen, B., Lowry, R., Chyen, D., Whittle, L., Thornton, J., Lim, C., Bradford, D., Yamakawa, Y., Leon, M., Brener, N., and Ethier, K.A. (2018). Youth risk behavior surveillance—United States, 2017. *Morbidity and Mortality Weekly Report Surveillance Summaries, 67*(8).

Kavuluru, R., Han, S., and Hahn, E.J. (2019). On the popularity of the USB flash drive-shaped electronic cigarette JUUL. *Tobacco Control, 28*(1), 110–112.

Kearney, M.S., and Levine, P.B. (2012). Why is the teen birth rate in the United States so high and why does it matter? *Journal of Economic Perspectives, 26*(2), 141–163.

Kearney, M.S., and Levine, P.B. (2015). Media influences on social outcomes: The impact of MTV's 16 and Pregnant on teen childbearing. *American Economic Review, 105*(12), 3597–3632.

King, B.M., Marino, L.E., and Barry, K.R. (2018). Does the Centers for Disease Control and Prevention's Youth Risk Behavior Survey underreport risky sexual behavior? *Sexually Transmitted Diseases, 45*(3), e10–e11.

Knoll, L.J., Magis-Weinberg, L., Speekenbrink, M., and Blakemore, S-J. (2015). Social influence on risk perception during adolescence. *Psychological Science, 26*(5), 583–592.

Kost, K., Maddow-Zimet, I., and Arpaia, A. (2017). *Pregnancies, Births and Abortions among Adolescents and Young Women in the United States, 2013: National and State Trends by Age, Race and Ethnicity.* New York, NY: Guttmacher Institute.

Langton, C.E. and Berger, L.M. (2011). Family structure and adolescent physical health, behavior, and emotional well-being. *Social Services Review, 85*(3), 323–357.

Lee, Y-K., Chang, C-T., Lin, Y., and Cheng, Z-H. (2014). The dark side of smartphone usage: Psychological traits, compulsive behavior and technostress. *Computers in Human Behavior, 31*, 373–383.

Lenhart, A., and Duggan, M. (2014). *Couples, the Internet, and Social Media.* Washington, DC: Pew Research Center.

Leventhal, T., Dupéré, V., and Brooks-Gunn, J. (2009). Neighborhood influences on adolescent development. In R.M. Lerner, and L. Steinberg (Eds.), *Handbook of Adolescent Psychology* (vol. 2, pp. 411–443). Hoboken, NJ: John Wiley & Sons, Inc.

Lindberg, L.D., Santelli, J.S., and Desai, S. (2016). Understanding the decline in adolescent fertility in the United States, 2007–2012. *Journal of Adolescent Health, 59*(5), 577–583.

Lindberg, L.D., Santelli, J.S., and Desai, S. (2018). Changing patterns of contraceptive use and the decline in rates of pregnancy and birth among U.S. adolescents, 2007–2014. *Journal of Adolescent Health, 63*(2), 253–256.

Livingston, G. (2018). *The Changing Profile of Unmarried Parents.* Washington, DC: Pew Research Center.

Lopez-Quintero, C., de los Cobos, J.P., Hasin, D.S., Okuda, M., Wang, S., Grant, B.F., and Blanco, C. (2011). Probability and predictors of transition from first use to dependence on nicotine, alcohol, cannabis, and cocaine: Results of the National Epidemiologic Survey on Alcohol and Related Conditions (NESARC). *Drug and Alcohol Dependence, 115*(1–2), 120–130.

Lugo-Gil, J., Lee, A., Vohra, D., Harding, J., Ochoa, L., and Goesling, B. (2018). *Updated Findings from the HHS Teen Pregnancy Prevention Evidence Review: August 2015 through October 2016.* Washington, DC: U.S. Department of Health and Human Services.

Mantey, D.S., Cooper, M.R., Clendennen, S.L., Pasch, K.E., and Perry, C.L. (2016). E-cigarette marketing exposure is associated with e-cigarette use among U.S. youth. *Journal of Adolescent Health, 58*(6), 686–690.

Mantey, D.S., Barroso, C.S., Kelder, B.T., and Kelder, S.H. (2019). Retail access to e-cigarettes and frequency of e-cigarette use in high school students. *Tobacco Regulatory Science, 5*(3), 280–290.

Martin, J.A., Hamilton, B.E., Osterman, M.J.K., Driscoll, A.K., and Drake, P. (2018). Births: Final data for 2017. *National Vital Statistics Reports, 67*(8), 1–50.

Markkula, J., Härkänen, T., and Raitasalo, K. (2019). Drunken driving and riding with a drunken driver: Adolescent types at higher risk. *Drugs: Education, Prevention and Policy*, 1–8.

Mashhoon, Y., Betts, J., Farmer, S.L., and Lukas, S.E. (2018). Early onset tobacco cigarette smokers exhibit deficits in response inhibition and sustained attention. *Drug and Alcohol Dependence, 184,* 48–56.

Maslowsky, J., Owotomo, O., Huntley, E.D., and Keating, D. (2019). Adolescent risk behavior: Differentiating reasoned and reactive risk-taking. *Journal of Youth and Adolescence, 48*(2), 243–255.

McKelvey, K., Baiocchi, M., and Halpern-Felsher, B. (2018). Adolescents' and young adults' use and perceptions of pod-based electronic cigarettes. *Journal of the American Medical Association Network Open, 1*(6), e183535.

McNeely, C. and Blanchard, J. (2010). *The Teen Years Explained: A Guide to Healthy Adolescent Development.* Baltimore, MD: Johns Hopkins Bloomberg School of Public Health, Center for Adolescent Health.

McWhirter, B.T., McWhirter, E.H., McWhirter, J.J., and McWhirter, R.J. (2013). *At-Risk Youth: A Comprehensive Response for Counsellors, Teachers, Psychologists, and Human Services Professionals.* Belmont, CA: Thompson Brooks/Cole.

Meisel, S.N. and Colder, C.R. (2019). Adolescent social norms and alcohol use: Separating between- and within-person associations to test reciprocal determinism. *Journal of Research on Adolescence.* Available: https://doi.org/10.1111/jora.12494.

Meyers, M.J., Delucchi, K., and Halpern-Felsher, B. (2017). Access to tobacco among California high school students: The role of family members, peers, and retail venues. *Journal of Adolescent Health, 61*(3), 385–388.

Morain, S.R. and Malek, J. (2017). Minimum age of sale for tobacco products and electronic cigarettes: Ethical acceptability of U.S. "tobacco 21 laws." *American Journal of Public Health, 107*(9), 1401–1405.

Moreno, M.A., and Whitehill, J.M. (2014). Influence of social media on alcohol use in adolescents and young adults. *Alcohol Research: Current Reviews, 36*(1), 91.

Murthy, V.H. (2017). E-cigarette use among youth and young adults: A major public health concern. *Journal of the American Medical Association Pediatrics, 171*(3), 209–210.

Murty, V.P., Calabro, F., and Luna, B. (2016). The role of experience in adolescent cognitive development: Integration of executive, memory, and mesolimbic systems. *Neuroscience & Biobehavioral Reviews, 70,* 46–58.

MyVoice. (2019). *Youth Perspectives on Being Healthy and Thriving.* Report commissioned by the Committee on Applying Lessons of Optimal Adolescent Health to Improve Behavioral Outcomes for Youth. Available: https://www.nap.edu/resource/25552/Youth%20 Perspectives%20on%20Being%20Healthy%20and%20Thriving.pdf.

National Academies of Sciences, Engineering, and Medicine (NASEM). (2016). *Preventing Bullying Through Science, Policy, and Practice.* Washington, DC: The National Academies Press.

———. (2017). *Community Violence as a Population Health Issue: Proceedings of a Workshop.* Washington, DC: The National Academies Press.

———. (2018a). *Violence and Mental Health: Opportunities for Prevention and Early Detection: Proceedings of a Workshop.* Washington, DC: The National Academies Press.

———. (2018b). *Public Health Consequences of E-cigarettes.* Washington, DC: The National Academies Press.

———. (2019). *The Promise of Adolescence: Realizing Opportunity for All Youth.* Washington, DC: The National Academies Press.

National Research Council and Institute of Medicine. (2004). *Reducing Underage Drinking: A Collective Responsibility.* Washington, DC: The National Academies Press.

Nguyen, N., McKelvey, K., and Halpern-Felsher, B. (2019). Popular flavors used in alternative tobacco products among young adults. *Journal of Adolescent Health, 65*(2), 306–308.

O'Dea, B., and Campbell, A. (2011). Healthy connections: Online social networks and their potential for peer support. *Studies in Health Technology and Informatics, 168*, 133–140.

Odgers, C.L., Robins, S.J., and Russell, M.A. (2010). Morbidity and mortality risk among the "forgotten few": Why are girls in the justice system in such poor health? *Law and Human Behavior, 34*(6), 429–444.

Odom, S.L., Thompson, J.L., Hedges, S., Boyd, B.A., Dykstra, J.R., Duda, M.A., Szidon, K.L., Smith, L.E., and Bord, A. (2015). Technology-aided interventions and instruction for adolescents with autism spectrum disorder. *Journal of Autism and Developmental Disorders, 45*(12), 3805–3819.

O'Donnell, M.P. (2017). *Health Promotion in the Workplace* (5th ed.). Troy, MI: Art & Science of Health Promotion Institute.

O'Keeffe, G.S., and Clarke-Pearson, K. (2011). The impact of social media on children, adolescents, and families. *Pediatrics, 127*(4), 800–804.

Paschall, M.J., Lipperman-Kreda, S., and Grube, J.W. (2014). Effects of the local alcohol environment on adolescents' drinking behaviors and beliefs. *Addiction, 109*(3), 407–416.

Peake, S.J., Dishion, T.J., Stormshak, E.A., Moore, W.E., and Pfeifer, J.H. (2013). Risk-taking and social exclusion in adolescence: Neural mechanisms underlying peer influences on decision-making. *Neuroimage, 82*, 23–34.

Peck, B., Manning, J., Tri, A., Skrzypczynski, D., Summers, M., and Grubb, K. (2016). What do people mean when they say they "had sex"? Connecting communication and behavior. In J. Manning and C. Noland (Eds.), *Contemporary Studies of Sexuality & Communication: Theoretical and Applied Perspectives* (pp. 3–13). Dubuque, IA: Kendall Hunt.

Penman-Aguilar, A., Carter, M., Snead, M.C., and Kourtis, A.P. (2013). Socioeconomic disadvantage as a social determinant of teen childbearing in the U.S. *Public Health Reports, 128* (Suppl 1), 5–22.

Pepper, J.K., Ribisl, K.M., and Brewer, N.T. (2016). Adolescents' interest in trying flavoured e-cigarettes. *Tobacco Control, 25*(Suppl 2), ii62–ii66.

Perikleous, E.P., Steiropoulos, P., Paraskakis, E., Constantinidis, T.C., and Nena, E. (2018). E-cigarette use among adolescents: An overview of the literature and future perspectives. *Frontiers in Public Health, 6*, 86.

Reyna, V.F. (2012). A new intuitionism: Meaning, memory, and development in fuzzy-trace theory. *Judgment and Decision Making, 7*(3), 332–359.

Roditis, M., Delucchi, K., Cash, D., and Halpern-Felsher, B. (2016). Adolescents' perceptions of health risks, social risks, and benefits differ across tobacco products. *Journal of Adolescent Health, 58*(5), 558–566.

Romer, D. (2010). Adolescent risk taking, impulsivity, and brain development: Implications for prevention. *Developmental Psychobiology, 52*(3), 263–276.

Romer, D., Reyna, V.F., and Satterthwaite, T.D. (2017). Beyond stereotypes of adolescent risk taking: Placing the adolescent brain in developmental context. *Developmental Cognitive Neuroscience, 27*, 19–34.

Ross, V., Jongen, E., Brijs, T., Ruiter, R., Brijs, K., and Wets, G. (2015). The relation between cognitive control and risky driving in young novice drivers. *Applied Neuropsychology, 22*(1), 61–72.

Sanders, S.A., and Reinisch, J.M. (1999). Would you say you had sex if...? *Journal of the American Medical Association, 281*(3), 275–277.

Sandfort, T.G.M., Orr, M., Hirsch, J.S., and Santelli, J. (2008). Long-term health correlates of timing of sexual debut: Results from a national U.S. study. *American Journal of Public Health, 98*(1), 155–161.

Santelli, J.S., Lindberg, L.D., Finer, L.B., and Singh, S. (2007). Explaining recent declines in adolescent pregnancy in the United States: The contribution of abstinence and improved contraceptive use. *American Journal of Public Health*, 97(1), 150–156.

Santelli, J., Sandfort, T., and Orr, M. (2008). Transnational comparisons of adolescent contraceptive use: What can we learn from these comparisons? *Archives of Pediatrics and Adolescent Medicine*, 162(1), 92–94.

Santelli, J.S., Kantor, L.M., Grilo, S.A., Speizer, I.S., Lindberg, L.D., Heitel, J., Schalet, A.T., Lyon, M.E., Mason-Jones, A.J., McGovern, T., Heck, C.J., Rogers, J., and Ott, M.A. (2017). Abstinence-only-until-marriage: An updated review of U.S. policies and programs and their impact. *Journal of Adolescent Health*, 61(3), 273–280.

Schaefer, D.R., Adams, J., and Haas, S.A. (2013). Social networks and smoking: Exploring the effects of peer influence and smoker popularity through simulations. *Health Education & Behavior*, 40(Suppl 1), 24s–32s.

Seemiller, C., and Grace, M. (2018). *Generation Z: A Century in the Making*. Abingdon, UK: Routledge.

Sherman, L.E., Payton, A.A., Hernandez, L.M., Greenfield, P.M., and Dapretto, M. (2016). The power of the like in adolescence: Effects of peer influence on neural and behavioral responses to social media. *Psychological Science*, 27(7), 1027–1035.

Sieving, R.E., McRee, A-L., McMorris, B.J., Shlafer, R.J., Gower, A.L., Kapa, H.M., Beckman, K.J., Doty, J.L., Plowman, S.L., and Resnick, M.D. (2017). Youth-adult connectedness: A key protective factor for adolescent health. *American Journal of Preventive Medicine*, 52(3s3), s275–s278.

Siqueira, L., and Smith, V.C. (2015). Binge drinking. *Pediatrics*, 136(3), e718–e726.

Sleiman, M., Logue, J.M., Montesinos, V.N., Russell, M.L., Litter, M.I., Gundel, L.A., and Destaillats, H. (2016). Emissions from electronic cigarettes: Key parameters affecting the release of harmful chemicals. *Environmental Science & Technology*, 50(17), 9644–9651.

Smit, K., Voogt, C., Hiemstra, M., Kleinjan, M., Otten, R., and Kuntsche, E. (2018). Development of alcohol expectancies and early alcohol use in children and adolescents: A systematic review. *Clinical Psychology Review*, 60, 136–146.

Smith, A.R., Chein, J., and Steinberg, L. (2013). Impact of socio-emotional context, brain development, and pubertal maturation on adolescent risk-taking. *Hormones and Behavior*, 64(2), 323–332.

Smith, A.R., Chein, J., and Steinberg, L. (2014). Peers increase adolescent risk taking even when the probabilities of negative outcomes are known. *Developmental Psychology*, 50(5), 1564–1568.

Smith, L.A., and Foxcroft, D.R. (2009). The effect of alcohol advertising, marketing and portrayal on drinking behaviour in young people: Systematic review of prospective cohort studies. *BMC Public Health*, 9(1), 51.

Squeglia, L.M., Rinker, D.A., Bartsch, H., Castro, N., Chung, Y., Dale, A.M., Jernigan, T.L., and Tapert, S.F. (2014). Brain volume reductions in adolescent heavy drinkers. *Developmental Cognitive Neuroscience*, 9, 117–125.

Stanwick, R. (2015). E-cigarettes: Are we renormalizing public smoking? Reversing five decades of tobacco control and revitalizing nicotiny dependency in children and youth in Canada. *Paediatrics & Child Health*, 20(2), 101–105.

Suleiman, A.B., Galván, A., Harden, K.P., and Dahl, R.E. (2017). Becoming a sexual being: The "elephant in the room" of adolescent brain development. *Developmental Cognitive Neuroscience*, 25, 209–220.

Telzer, E.H., Fuligni, A.J., Lieberman, M.D., Miernicki, M.E., and Galvan, A. (2015). The quality of adolescents' peer relationships modulates neural sensitivity to risk taking. *Social Cognitive and Affective Neuroscience*, 10(3), 389–398.

Thapa, A., Cohen, J., Guffey, S., and Higgins-D'Alessandro, A. (2013). A review of school climate research. *Review of Educational Research, 83*(3), 357–385.

Tolman, D.L., and McClelland, S.I. (2011). Normative sexuality development in adolescence: A decade in review, 2000–2009. *Journal of Research on Adolescence, 21*(1), 242–255.

Tolou-Shams, M., Harrison, A., Hirschtritt, M.E., Dauria, E., and Barr-Walker, J. (2019). Substance use and HIV among justice-involved youth: Intersecting risks. *Current HIV/AIDS Reports, 16*(1), 37–47.

Tsai, K.M., Telzer, E.H., and Fuligni, A.J. (2013). Continuity and discontinuity in perceptions of family relationships from adolescence to young adulthood. *Child Development, 84*(2), 471–484.

Tulloch, T., and Kaufman, M. (2013). Adolescent sexuality. *Pediatrics in Review, 34*(1), 29–37.

U.S. Department of Health and Human Services (HHS). (2012). *Preventing Tobacco Use among Youth and Young Adults: A Report of the Surgeon General.* Atlanta, GA: Centers for Disease Control and Prevention, National Center for Chronic Disease Prevention and Health Promotion, Office on Smoking and Health.

———. (2014). *The Health Consequences of Smoking: 50 Years of Progress: A Report of the Surgeon General.* Atlanta, GA: Centers for Disease Control and Prevention, National Center for Chronic Disease Prevention and Health Promotion, Office on Smoking and Health.

———. (2016a). *E-cigarette Use Among Youth and Young Adults: A Report of the Surgeon General.* Atlanta, GA: Centers for Disease Control and Prevention, National Center for Chronic Disease Prevention and Health Promotion, Office on Smoking and Health.

———. (2016b). *Facing Addiction in America: The Surgeon General's Report on Alcohol, Drugs, and Health.* Washington, DC: Office of the Surgeon General.

———. (2017a). *Report to Congress on the Prevention and Reduction of Underage Drinking.* Rockville, MD: Substance Use and Mental Health Services Administration.

———. (2017b). *Underage Drinking Fact Sheet.* Bethesda, MD: National Institutes of Health, National Institute on Alcohol Abuse and Alcoholism.

———. (2018a). *Adolescent Health: Think, Act, Grow® Playbook.* Washington, DC: Office of Population Affairs, Office of Adolescent Health.

———. (2018b). *Surgeon General's Advisory on E-cigarette Use among Youth.* Atlanta, GA: Centers for Disease Control and Prevention, National Center for Chronic Disease Prevention and Health Promotion, Office on Smoking and Health.

U.S. Department of Transportation. (2019). *1999–2017 Young Drivers Traffic Safety Fact Sheets.* Available: https://crashstats.nhtsa.dot.gov.

U.S. Food and Drug Administration. (2018a). *Statement from FDA Commissioner Scott Gottlieb, MD, on New Steps to Address Epidemic of Youth E-cigarette Use.* Available: https://www.fda.gov/news-events/press-announcements/statement-fda-commissioner-scott-gottlieb-md-new-steps-address-epidemic-youth-e-cigarette-use.

U.S. Food and Drug Administration. (2018b). *Statement from FDA Commissioner Scott Gottlieb, MD, on Proposed New Steps to Protect Youth by Preventing Access to Flavored Tobacco Products and Banning Menthol in Cigarettes.* Available: https://www.fda.gov/news-events/press-announcements/statement-fda-commissioner-scott-gottlieb-md-proposed-new-steps-protect-youth-preventing-access.

van den Bos, W., and Hertwig, R. (2017). Adolescents display distinctive tolerance to ambiguity and to uncertainty during risky decision making. *Scientific Reports, 7,* 40962.

Vassoler, F.M., and Sadri-Vakili, G. (2014). Mechanisms of transgenerational inheritance of addictive-like behaviors. *Neuroscience, 264,* 198–206.

Vermeersch, H., T'Sjoen, G., Kaufman, J-M., and Vincke, J. (2008). The role of testosterone in aggressive and non-aggressive risk-taking in adolescent boys. *Hormones and Behavior, 53*(3), 463–471.

Wang, B., King, B.A., Corey, C.G., Arrazola, R.A., and Johnson, S.E. (2014). Awareness and use of non-conventional tobacco products among U.S. students, 2012. *American Journal of Preventive Medicine, 47*(2 Suppl 1), S36–S52.

Warner, T.D., Giordano, P.C., Manning, W.D., and Longmore, M.A. (2011). Everybody's doin' it (right?): Neighborhood norms and sexual activity in adolescence. *Social Science Research, 40*(6), 1676–1690.

Wellman, R.J., Dugas, E.N., Dutczak, H., O'Loughlin, E.K., Datta, G.D., Lauzon, B., and O'Loughlin, J. (2016). Predictors of the onset of cigarette smoking: A systematic review of longitudinal population-based studies in youth. *American Journal of Preventive Medicine, 51*(5), 767–778.

Willett, J.G., Bennett, M., Hair, E.C., Xiao, H., Greenberg, M.S., Harvey, E., Cantrell, J., and Vallone, D. (2019). Recognition, use and perceptions of JUUL among youth and young adults. *Tobacco Control, 28*(1), 115–116.

Wilson, S.J., Tanner-Smith, E.E., Lipsey, M.W., Steinka-Fry, K., and Morrison, J. (2011). Dropout prevention and intervention programs: Effects on school completion and dropout among school aged children and youth. *Campbell Systematic Reviews, 8*, 61.

Wood, A.P., Dawe, S., and Gullo, M.J. (2013). The role of personality, family influences, and prosocial risk-taking behavior on substance use in early adolescence. *Journal of Adolescence, 36*(5), 871–881.

World Health Organization. (2017). *WHO Report on the Global Tobacco Epidemic, 2017: Monitoring Tobacco Use and Prevention Policies* (No. 9241512822). Geneva, Switzerland: Author.

Wu, J., Witkiewitz, K., McMahon, R.J., and Dodge, K.A. (2010). A parallel process growth mixture model of conduct problems and substance use with risky sexual behavior. *Drug and Alcohol Dependence, 111*(3), 207–214.

4

Core Components of Programs Focused on Optimal Health

[My school] could provide social situations that could teach you important things like establishing boundaries, how to work with other people, and how to handle social situations.

Female, age 17[1]

As described in Chapter 1, the committee was charged with identifying the *key elements* or *core components* of programs that may be successful in preventing risk behaviors and improving outcomes for youth using an optimal health lens. In particular, the sponsor was interested in using a core components methodology to align with work on other current federal research and evaluation initiatives (Blase and Fixsen, 2013). This chapter describes the committee's approach to this task. First, we provide a brief description of the core components approach. We then describe the methods we used to identify and summarize the evidence on core components of adolescent health programs. Finally, we describe the results of our systematic review and the findings from a complementary review of papers that use a core components approach.

---

[1]Response to MyVoice survey question: "Specifically, what could your school do to help you live your best life (now or in the past)?" See the discussion of the MyVoice methodology in Appendix B for more detail.

THE CORE COMPONENTS APPROACH TO
EVIDENCE-BASED PRACTICE

Core program or intervention components are discrete, reliably identifiable techniques, strategies, or practices that are intended to influence the behavior, outcomes, or well-being of a service recipient (Blase and Fixsen, 2013). Core components may reflect aspects of intervention *content,* defined as specific knowledge or actions thought to influence behavior (e.g., communication skills); the *processes,* methods, or techniques through which service providers deliver content components and support the behavior change process (e.g., modeling); the *locations* and *formats* that make up the intervention delivery circumstances; and the *implementation strategies* used to facilitate intervention delivery (e.g., provider training, availability of manuals). In this report, we use the term *core components* to refer to any of these aspects of interventions, although other terms are also used to refer to this family of approaches to evidence-based practice, including *common elements, kernels,* and *core practice elements* (Barth and Liggett-Creel, 2014; Chorpita, Delaiden, and Weisz, 2005; Embry and Biglan, 2008; Hogue et al., 2017). In general, these approaches share being based on the idea that interventions comprise discrete components that can be identified, organized, and combined in different ways to achieve the intended results.

Core components approaches have emerged as a complement to the common approach to evidence-based programs (EBPs) that focuses on identifying distinct model programs that have demonstrated positive impacts. Such model programs usually have a brand name (e.g., Reducing the Risk, Positive Action, Be Proud! Be Responsible!), are generally accompanied by a program manual, and sometimes offer training or certification by the program developer. These programs typically receive the "evidence-based" designation as a result of at least one experimental or quasi-experimental study that demonstrates a statistically significant positive impact on an outcome of interest. Registries such as Blueprints for Healthy Youth Development[2] review the research on candidate programs and provide listings of those that meet their evidence standards. More recently, tiered evidence schemes and some federal grant funding have begun mandating or incentivizing the use of model programs.

While the evidence backing model programs is derived from some of the highest-quality research available, the focus on EBPs has several drawbacks. First, often only one or, at best, a few studies of a program have assessed its impact, leaving open the question of generalizability. Second, this approach implies that the program must be implemented with fidelity

---

[2]For more information, see https://www.blueprintsprograms.org.

to the original model to achieve similar results, which requires significant training of facilitators and inhibits what might be effective local adaptations. Finally, most programs already in operation are likely to be reluctant to abandon their current practice to adopt something new because of cost, provider resistance to change, contractual obligations, local support for the current program, or other factors (Blase and Fixsen, 2013).

Core components approaches to EBPs seek to address some of these drawbacks. For example, because core components approaches unpack programs into discrete components and often examine aspects of their delivery format, dosage, implementation strategies, and delivery personnel, they afford more flexibility or creativity in what and how services are delivered. In an environment of limited resources and competing priorities, such flexibility may promote more widespread adoption of effective practices. Because aspects of adolescent health overlap and are interrelated, core components approaches also offer an efficient strategy for supporting multiple aspects of youth development.

Recent research has shown the utility of this approach for adolescent opioid use disorder (OUD), as well as youth program management and quality improvement. For instance, researchers at the Center on Addiction were able to identify 21 core techniques focused on family psychoeducation, medication options, and shared decision making that were most effective in adolescent OUD treatment (National Academies of Sciences, Engineering, and Medicine [NASEM], 2019). Additionally, the David P. Weikart Center for Youth Program Quality (2019) used this approach to identify high-quality practices for after-school programs, which led to the development of the Youth Program Quality Assessment (NASEM, 2019).

As the use of core components approaches to EBPs has spread, a variety of methodologies for identifying such components have emerged. For example, the distillation and matching method focuses on identifying and distilling key practices from program manuals and then matching those practices to particular client needs (Chorpita and Daleiden, 2009; Chorpita, Delaiden, and Weisz, 2005). Embry and Biglan's (2008) kernels method relies on evidence from peer-reviewed experimental studies to identify practices that can be delivered alone or in combination or added on to existing programs. More recently, adaptive research designs have emerged that can provide an analytic strategy for identifying core components (Pallmann et al., 2018). Other approaches to identifying core components involve systematic reviews of evidence, meta-analyses, or reviews of systematic reviews or meta-analyses (Boustani et al., 2015; Lipsey, 2018; Peters et al., 2009).

THE COMMITTEE'S APPROACH

Strategy

The committee's primary strategy involved a systematic review of systematic reviews and meta-analyses, conducted in April 2019. We considered other approaches, including a meta-analysis of primary studies; however, such a task was not possible within the time constraints for this consensus study. The approach we took enabled examination of the largest possible body of evidence in the available time.

To supplement our systematic review, we examined research papers focused on identifying and integrating the core components of effective youth programs. More specifically, the purpose of this secondary strategy was to (1) provide additional evidence in support of or in contrast to the core components identified in our systematic review, and (2) find any additional core components not previously identified.

Eligibility Criteria

To identify the most relevant systematic reviews and meta-analyses for our review, stay within the scope of the charge in our statement of task, and ensure that the articles we reviewed met minimum quality standards for systematic reviews and meta-analyses, we used a set of eligibility criteria to determine which documents would be eligible for this review. These criteria were informed by the scoring methods used by the U.S. Department of Justice's Office of Justice Programs (2013) to analyze programs and practices as part of its CrimeSolutions.gov initiative. Our set of criteria is described below.

Type of review. To be eligible, a manuscript must have been clearly described as a systematic review or meta-analysis and to have evidence of peer review. Narrative literature reviews were not eligible for our systematic review.

Literature search. The literature search that guided the inclusion of primary studies in a meta-analysis or systematic review must have included at least two sources and must have provided evidence that unpublished literature was sought in the search.

Intervention. A meta-analysis or systematic review must have included at least two studies of the practice of interest, as defined below under the criterion "primary aim of the intervention."

Aggregation. If there was a meta-analysis, it must have aggregated the results from at least two studies.

Primary aim of the intervention. The programs included in a meta-analysis or systematic review had to address behaviors and outcomes in one of the five dimensions of optimal health on which this report focuses.[3] Reviews that included programs targeting risk behaviors or negative outcomes relating to the optimal health dimensions (e.g., substance use, sexual behavior) were also eligible.

1. *Physical health.* Two aspects of physical health were prioritized for the review.
   — *Substance use.* A meta-analysis or systematic review must have focused on prevention or intervention programs intended to prevent or reduce tobacco use (including e-cigarettes), alcohol use, or illicit drug use.[4] Programs could be educational, skill-building, or psychosocial. Primary, secondary, and tertiary prevention programs were eligible. Medical intervention or treatment programs were excluded because they were not generalizable or representative of the broader youth population.
   — *Pregnancy prevention/sexual health and/or reproductive health.* A meta-analysis or systematic review must have covered programs intended to reduce teenage pregnancy, sexually transmitted infections (STIs), or related sexual risk behaviors through educational, skill-building, and/or psychosocial intervention or programming. Primary, secondary, and tertiary prevention programs were eligible.
2. *Emotional health.* A meta-analysis or systematic review must have included interventions targeting resilience, mental or emotional health, stress management, emotion regulation, or self-regulation.
3. *Social health.* A meta-analysis or systematic review must have included interventions targeting social-emotional learning, conflict resolution, assertiveness, or social skills.
4. *Intellectual health.* A meta-analysis or systematic review must have included interventions broadly targeting academic achievement, academic performance, or learning, including academic programs, after-school programs, and mentoring.
5. *Spiritual health.* A meta-analysis or systematic review must have included interventions targeting mindfulness, character education, or moral or spiritual development.

---

[3]The five dimensions of optimal health are broad and cover many aspects of adolescent health and development. The committee selected several topics within each of these broad categories that are of particular relevance to healthy adolescent development.

[4]Although the committee specifically targeted tobacco and alcohol use in this report, illicit drug use was included in the search criteria since many substance use programs for tobacco and alcohol also target illicit drugs. However, "illicit drugs" were rarely defined or disaggregated in these studies, so a focus on specific illicit drugs was not possible in this report.

Primary outcomes. A meta-analysis or systematic review must have reported on at least one of the following eligible outcomes related to the dimensions of optimal adolescent health that are the focus of this report:

- sexual activity, including sexual initiation, frequency, and number of partners;
- contraceptive use, including condom use;
- pregnancy;
- STIs;
- behavioral intentions regarding use of substances, including tobacco, alcohol, and illicit drugs;
- substance use or misuse, including frequency or quantity of use, type of use, use/no use, time since last use, etc., and encompassing use of tobacco, alcohol, and illicit drugs alone or in combination;
- social skills or social-emotional skills;
- mental health, reduced stress, resilience, and self-regulation;
- academic achievement or performance; and
- mindfulness, moral development, and religiosity.

Age of samples. Samples included in a meta-analysis or systematic review were restricted to adolescents ages 10–19. If a sample combined adolescents with adults, the results for the youth must have been reported separately.

Control groups. All studies included in a meta-analysis or systematic review had to include an appropriate control, comparison, or counter-factual condition, or the meta-analysis or systematic review must have analyzed those studies without appropriate comparison conditions separately from those with appropriate counterfactuals.

Single group. A meta-analysis or systematic review could include pre–post or head-to-head comparison studies, but these must have been separated from those with comparison groups.

Specialized sample. A meta-analysis or systematic review must not have been conducted on narrowly focused samples of adolescents, including but not limited to those with diagnosed medical conditions (e.g., chronic physical disability or disease, mental health condition).

Reporting of results. A meta-analysis or systematic review must have reported effect sizes that represent the magnitude of the treatment effect.

Combining effect sizes. When an average effect size was reported for multiple studies, all effect sizes in the combination must have addressed the same type of relationship.

Publication date. At least 50 percent of the studies included in a meta-analysis or systematic review must have been published or otherwise available in or after 1980.

Publication location. The studies in a meta-analysis or systematic review must not have been conducted exclusively in low- or middle-income countries or be single-country studies other than in the United States (e.g., meta-analyses of research conducted entirely in Spanish locations were not eligible).

Results of Literature Search

Using the above eligibility criteria as a guide, the committee conducted a comprehensive literature search to identify relevant studies. We searched the following electronic bibliographic databases for articles published between 2009 and 2019: Cochrane Database of Systematic Reviews, Campbell Collaboration Library, PubMed, and PsycINFO. Also included were meta-analyses and systematic reviews meeting our criteria that were recommended by committee members, by individuals attending our public information-gathering session, and by members of the public.

The search terms were adapted to each database, and separate searches were conducted around the different domains of optimal adolescent health. Generally, three blocks of terms were used: one block describing the sample or population of interest (e.g., teens, adolescents), one block describing the optimal adolescent health domain or subdomain of interest (e.g., sexual risk behavior, pregnancy), and one block identifying meta-analyses and systematic reviews. Our full search strategy is detailed in Appendix A.

Once potential articles had been identified, committee members screened the titles and abstracts of all of these articles for relevance to this review. The full-text versions of all articles deemed relevant based on the title and abstract screening were then evaluated by two committee members against the full eligibility criteria. Conflicts were resolved by consensus. The title/abstract screening and full eligibility review were conducted using Covidence systematic review software (Veritas Health Innovation, 2019).

These procedures resulted in the identification of 31 meta-analyses and systematic reviews. Figure 4-1 shows the flow of manuscripts through the search and screening process using the preferred reporting items for systematic reviews and meta-analyses (PRISMA) guidelines (Moher et al., 2009).

Eighteen of the 31 articles were focused on the domain of physical health, which was further subdivided into articles focused on substance use (n = 10) and sexual health (n = 8).[5,6] Another 6 articles focused on

---

[5]Although many adolescent behaviors and outcomes fall under physical health (e.g., eating, obesity), the committee's review focused on substance use (alcohol and tobacco, as well as other drugs when combined with alcohol or tobacco) and sexual health, as described in Chapter 3 and in the search and exclusion criteria noted above.

[6]Three papers that report on the same data or study as other articles were used to supplement study information but were not included in this count.

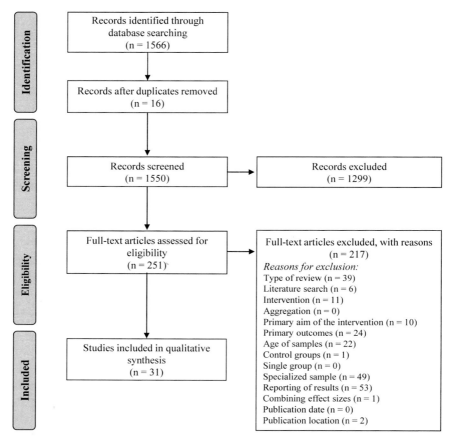

FIGURE 4-1 From a database search that yielded 1,565 articles, the committee identified 31 that met its criteria for review.

NOTES: Articles with ineligible publication dates were excluded during the screening process.

Three articles reported on the same set of papers as another eligible study and were considered together as one review in the qualitative synthesis.

SOURCE: Adapted from PRISMA reporting guidelines (Moher et al., 2009).

outcomes related to emotional health. One article focused on intellectual health. None of the studies identified in this review focused exclusively on social or spiritual health. The remaining articles considered a variety of behaviors and outcomes that mapped onto multiple optimal health domains (n = 6). Table 4-1 shows the articles that fell into each category.

TABLE 4-1 Articles Identified in the Systematic Review by Optimal Health Domains (n = 31)

Physical Health (n = 18)		Emotional Health (n = 6)	Social Health (n = 0)	Intellectual Health (n = 1)	Spiritual Health (n = 0)
Substance Use (n = 10)	Sexual Health (n = 8)				
• Carney et al. (2016) • Champion et al. (2013) • Faggiano et al. (2014) • Ferri et al. (2013) • Hodder et al. (2017) • MacArthur et al. (2016) • Onrust et al. (2016) • Tanner-Smith et al. (2015) • Thomas, Lorenzetti, and Spragins (2013) • Thomas, McLellan, and Perera (2015)	• Aslam et al. (2017)/ Whitaker et al. (2016)* • Chin et al. (2012) • DeSmet et al. (2015) • Harden et al. (2009) • Lopez et al. (2016) • Marseille et al. (2018) • Oringanje et al. (2016)/ Picot et al. (2012)/ Shepherd et al. (2010)*	• Calear and Christensen (2010) • Clarke, Kuosmanen, and Barry (2015) • Corrieri et al. (2014) • Das et al. (2016) • Dray et al. (2017) • van Genugten et al. (2017)		• Hahn et al. (2015)/ Wilson et al. (2011)*	

Multiple Optimal Health Areas (n = 6)

- Ciocanel et al. (2017)
- Durlak, Weissberg, and Pachan (2010)
- Durlak et al. (2011)
- Klingbeil et al. (2017)
- MacArthur et al. (2018)
- Taylor et al. (2017)

*Indicates two articles that were identified that were part of the same project and used the same set of studies for their manuscript, and were reviewed together.

Our inability to find studies that focused exclusively on social or spiritual health is reflected in the limitations of O'Donnell's (2009) optimal health definition (see Chapter 2). First, these dimensions of optimal health are much more difficult to measure than the physical, emotional, and intellectual domains, whose measurement can often rely on standardized tools or the presence/absence of a disease or condition. Second, the interdependence and interaction among the dimensions can make them difficult to disentangle. Accordingly, many programs incorporating social or spiritual health are categorized under "multiple optimal health domains."

Organizing Framework

The committee's methodological approach for extracting information from each article drew on the methods used by other core components researchers and was guided by the organizing framework illustrated in Figure 4-2. This framework represents the committee's consensus about the common features of programs and interventions targeting adolescent behavior. Beyond its utility for this report, the committee's framework provides an important structure for identifying what matters for promoting optimal adolescent health. Each of the areas identified in this framework is described in greater detail below.

Program Types

Program types were classified using the Institute of Medicine's (IOM, 1994) intervention classifications and the levels of prevention in the public health prevention framework (Katz and Ali, 2009) (see Figure 4-3).

Institute of Medicine (IOM) intervention classifications The IOM intervention classifications—universal, selective, and indicated—were based on those proposed by Gordon (1983). Universal interventions target an entire population, regardless of the members' levels of risk. Selective interventions are those that target a subset of the population that may be considered "at risk." Finally, indicated interventions are provided to those who are already beginning to experience the effects of a specific health outcome (Institute of Medicine, 1994).

Levels of prevention The committee chose to use the three-level public health prevention framework to guide its identification of programs and interventions (Katz and Ali, 2009). As noted in Chapter 1, the prevention framework is designed with health outcomes as the key target. Although a health behavior is an important predictor of a health outcome, behaviors

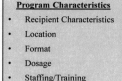
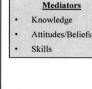

Program Types	Program Characteristics	Mediators	Targets
• IOM Intervention Classifications • Levels of Prevention	• Recipient Characteristics • Location • Format • Dosage • Staffing/Training • Delivery Mechanism • Optimal Health Domain-Based Content	• Knowledge • Attitudes/Beliefs • Skills	• Behaviors • Outcomes

FIGURE 4-2 Organizing framework based on the committee's consensus regarding the features of programs or interventions that have the potential to promote optimal adolescent health.

Program Types

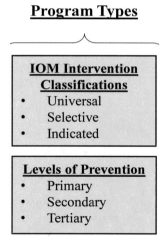

IOM Intervention Classifications
- Universal
- Selective
- Indicated

Levels of Prevention
- Primary
- Secondary
- Tertiary

FIGURE 4-3 Components included in program type.

are considered to be modifiable risk factors that are a focus in primary prevention activities rather than outcomes themselves.

In this model, *primary* prevention targets the risk factors for a disease or condition, with the intent of intervening before the disease or condition occurs. Included in primary prevention are vaccination and behavior change programs, both of which can prevent the onset or impact of the disease or condition (Centers for Disease Control and Prevention [CDC], 2017; U.S. Preventive Services Task Force, 2018). *Secondary* prevention focuses on early identification of high-risk populations, which can help slow or stop the progression of a disease or condition (CDC, 2017; U.S. Preventive Services Task Force, 2018). These activities may include early testing or monitoring for signs or symptoms of the disease or condition. *Tertiary* prevention encompasses treatment and rehabilitation after onset or diagnosis, which may prevent future incidence of the disease or condition (CDC, 2017; U.S. Preventive Services Task Force, 2018).

Program Characteristics

The committee identified a comprehensive list of characteristics that could describe the programs and interventions included in our review (see Figure 4-4). These characteristics were categorized by recipient character-

Program Characteristics

Recipient Characteristics
- Age (mean or range)
- Biological sex groups
- Racial/ethnic groups
- LGBTQ groups
- Other

Location
- School
- Home/ housing
- Faith-based
- Community
- Residential facility
- Online/computer
- Phone
- Primary care clinic
- Mental health clinic
- Other

Format
Group size
- Individualized
- Small group (<10)
- Large group (>10)
- Other

Method
- In-person
- Phone
- Online/computer
- Video
- Slides
- Other

Dosage
- Number of sessions
- Length of sessions

Staffing
- Teachers
- Parents/family
- Peers
- Social worker/counselor
- Primary care provider
- Mental health provider
- Researchers
- Graduate students
- Community health workers
- Mentors
- Faith-based
- Other

Training
- Trained/untrained
- Number of hours

Delivery Mechanism
- Information provision
- Behavioral rehearsal
- Game
- Demonstration
- Service provision
- Role play/practice
- Lecture
- Videos
- Discussion
- Test/quiz
- Homework/workbooks
- Other

Optimal Health Domain–Based Content

Physical
Sexual behavior
- Abstinence
- Risk reduction
- Risk discontinuation
- Anatomy/physiology
- Puberty/development
- Pregnancy/reproductive health
- Healthy relationships
- Personal safety/consent
- LGBTQ
- Contraception
  — Condoms
  — Hormonal methods
  — Other methods
- STI/STD/HIV
  — Information
  — Screening
  — Treatment
  — Vaccination
- Other

Substance use
- Type
  — Alcohol
  — Tobacco
  — Other drugs
- Abstinence
- Cessation
- Risk reduction
- Consent
- Brain development

Emotional
- Cognitive-behavioral therapy (CBT)
- Motivational interviewing
- Meditation
- Mindfulness
- Self-affirmation
- Self-esteem
- Other

Social
- Communication skills
- Conflict resolution/social problem solving
- Refusal skills
- Social influence/actual vs. perceived social norms
- Social support
- Social capital
- Social competence
- Other

Spiritual
- Morals/values
- Spirituality/religion
- Volunteering/civic engagement
- Goal setting
- Identity development
- Other

Intellectual
- School engagement/attendance
- Vocational/skills training
- College preparation
- School restructuring
- Supplemental academic services
- Alternative schooling
- Other

Multiple domains/Other:
- Positive youth development
- Contracting
- Rewards
- Punishment
- Natural consequences
- Action planning
- Comparisons or pro/con
- Case management
- Other

FIGURE 4-4 Components included in program characteristics.

istics, location, format, dosage, staffing, delivery mechanism, and optimal health domain–based content. Programs and interventions were not limited to one identifying characteristic per category. Recognizing that this list was not exhaustive, each category also included space for the identification of "other" characteristics that could emerge in the review.

Recipient characteristics   Recipient characteristics identified by the committee were age, biological sex, race/ethnicity, and sexual orientation/gender identity (LGBTQ). For age, either the range of ages or the mean age of recipients in the program or intervention needed to be 10–19 (see the discussion of eligibility criteria in the previous section). Biological sex, racial/ethnic, and LGBTQ group information was recorded to note whether an intervention was targeted to a particular demographic group (e.g., females only, black/African American adolescents).

Location   Location referred to the place where the program or intervention occurred. Locations could include schools; homes or housing; faith-based settings; community settings; residential facilities; online or on a computer; by phone; or in a clinic, such as a primary care or mental health provider office.

Format   Format included both group size and the method by which the program or intervention was delivered. Group sizes identified by the committee were individualized or one-on-one, small groups of fewer than 10 adolescents, and larger groups of 10 or more. Methods referred to how the intervention was provided, and included in-person, phone, online/computer-based, video, or slides.

Dosage   Dosage represented the amount of the program or intervention that was provided. Included in this category were the number and duration of sessions or programs.

Staffing   Program staffing referred to the person or people who delivered the program or intervention. The committee identified teachers, parents or family members, peers, social workers or counselors, primary care providers, mental health providers, researchers, graduate students, community health workers, mentors, and faith-based staff in the initial list. Staffing also referred to whether program staff were trained and if so, the number of training hours.

Delivery mechanism   Delivery mechanisms were the ways in which the material was delivered in the program or intervention. Delivery mechanisms identified by the committee included providing information, behavioral rehearsal, games, demonstrations, service provision, role play or practice, lectures, videos, discussions, tests or quizzes, and homework or workbooks.

Optimal Health Domain–Based Content

Content referred to the types of information, messages, or skills that the program sought to provide, enhance, or encourage. The committee identified a number of different types of content, which were further categorized by optimal health domain and, in the case of physical health, the behavior of interest. Again, understanding that this list was not exhaustive, we included space to identify any other content that was not on the initial list.

Physical health

- *Substance use.* Content for substance use included substance type (alcohol, tobacco, other drugs), abstinence messaging, cessation, risk reduction, consent, and brain development.
- *Sexual behavior.* Content for sexual health programs included abstinence messaging; risk reduction or risk discontinuation; anatomy and physiology; puberty and pubertal development; pregnancy and reproductive health; healthy relationships; personal safety and consent; sexual orientation and gender identity (LGBTQ); contraception (including condoms, hormonal methods, and other methods); and STI, sexually transmitted disease (STD), or HIV information, screening, treatment, and vaccination.

Emotional health   Emotional health–based content included cognitive-behavioral therapy–based techniques, motivational interviewing, meditation, mindfulness, self-affirmation, and self-esteem.

Social health   Content based in social health included communication skills, conflict resolution and social problem solving, refusal skills, social influences or social norms, social support, social capital, and social competence.

Spiritual health   Spiritual health content included morals and values, spirituality or religion, volunteering and civic engagement, goal setting, and identity development.

Intellectual health   Content in the intellectual health category included school engagement, vocational or skills training, college preparatory activities, school restructuring, supplemental academic services, and alternative schooling.

Multiple domains   Finally, there were a number of topics that did not fit into a single optimal health domain. These included positive youth development, contracting, rewards and punishments, natural consequences, action planning, making comparisons, and case management.

Mediators

Program or intervention mediators were the mechanisms or processes through which the targeted behaviors or outcomes were influenced (see Figure 4-5). The initial set of mediators identified by the committee included the knowledge, attitudes or beliefs, and skills that a program may promote, enhance, or encourage. Knowledge included providing information, while attitudes and beliefs included resilience, behavioral intentions, self-efficacy, and social norms. Most mediators were specific skills (i.e., knowing how and being able to do something), and were further categorized as social-emotional, refusal, prosocial behavior, mindfulness, attention, and cognitive flexibility.

Targets

The targets of programs were the behaviors and outcomes that each program sought to prevent or promote, and were categorized by optimal health domain (see Figure 4-6). In line with the levels of public health prevention framework, the outcomes were the conditions of interest, while the behaviors represented modifiable precursors for primary prevention activities.

Mediators

- Knowledge
  — Information
- Attitudes/Beliefs
  — Resilience
  — Intentions
  — Self-efficacy
  — Social norms
- Skills
  — Social-emotional
  — Refusal
  — Prosocial behavior
  — Mindfulness
  — Attention
  — Cognitive flexibility
- Other

FIGURE 4-5 Components included in mediators.

Targets

Behaviors

Physical

Sexual behavior
- Ever had sex
  - — Vaginal
  - — Oral
  - — Anal
- Frequency
- Current activity
- Partners
- Protection
  - — Condom use
  - — Contraception use
  - — Dual method use
- STI/HIV testing
- Other

Substance use
- Ever used
- Frequency
- Current use
- Binge/excessive use
- Other

Emotional

Internalizing
- Self-harm
- Suicidal ideation
- Suicide attempt
- Depressive symptoms
- Anxiety symptoms
- Stress
- Emotional distress
- Psychosomatization
- Self-esteem
- Psychological adjustment
- Other

Externalizing
- Delinquency
- Violence
- Conduct problems
- Other

Social
- Communication
- Conflict resolution
- Creating relationships
- Bullying
- Other

Spiritual
- Mindfulness
- Meditation
- Civic engagement
- Goal-setting
- Religious attendance
- Other

Intellectual
- Enrollment
- Attendance
- Academic adjustment/school bonding
- Other

Outcomes

Physical

Sexual behavior
- Romantic relationships
- Intimacy
- STI/STD/HIV
- Pregnancy
- Sexual assault/abuse
- Relationship based violence
- Other

Substance use
- Abuse
- Addiction
- Unintentional injury
- Disease/disability
- Death
- Other

Emotional

Internalizing
- Anxiety disorder
- Depression disorder
- Panic attack
- Suicide
- Other

Externalizing
- Arrest
- Intentional injury
- Unintentional injury
- Other

Social
- Relationships
- Isolation
- Other

Spiritual
- Identity
- Morals/values
- Other

Intellectual
- Grades
- Academic achievement
- School completion
- Other

FIGURE 4-6 Components included in targets.

Physical health

- *Substance use.* For each substance type, behaviors included ever using, frequency of use, current use, and binging or excessive use. The outcomes associated with substance use included substance abuse or addiction, unintentional injury, disease or disability, and death.
- *Sexual behavior.* Sexual behaviors included ever having sex (vaginal, oral, anal, or unspecified); sex frequency; current sexual activity; number of sexual partners; use of protection including condoms (for prevention of STI or pregnancy), contraception (pregnancy), or dual methods (STI and pregnancy); and STI or HIV testing. Sexual behavior outcomes were romantic relationships, intimacy, STIs/STDs/HIV, pregnancy, sexual assault or abuse, and relationship-based violence.

Emotional health   Although emotional health targets often have similar content, the behaviors and outcomes may differ, and are often categorized as internalizing or externalizing. *Internalizing* behaviors included self-harm, suicidal ideation, suicide attempt, depression symptoms, anxiety symptoms, stress, emotional distress, self-esteem, and psychological adjustment, while internalizing outcomes were anxiety or depression disorders, panic attacks, and suicide. *Externalizing* behaviors included delinquency, violence, and conduct problems, and externalizing outcomes were arrest, intentional injuries, and unintentional injuries.

Social health   Social health behaviors included communication, conflict resolution, creating relationships, and bullying. Outcomes were formed relationships and social inclusion.

Spiritual health   Spiritual health behaviors were mindfulness, meditation, civic engagement, goal setting, and religious attendance. Outcomes included established identity and moral or value systems.

Intellectual health   Intellectual health behaviors were school enrollment and attendance, and academic adjustment or school bonding. Associated outcomes included grades, academic achievements, and school completion.

RESULTS OF THE COMMITTEE'S SYSTEMATIC REVIEW

The committee examined several types of information from the eligible systematic reviews and meta-analyses, including the findings reported and any core components of the programs and interventions that were recorded or identified in the manuscripts. Most important, we carefully reviewed the moderator and subgroup analyses reported in each review in order to identify any core components with empirical support. The results of our systematic review of reviews and meta-analyses are summarized below by optimal health domain.

Physical Health

Substance Use

The committee reviewed 10 systematic reviews and meta-analyses that examined programs and interventions focused on prevention or reduction of youth substance use, including alcohol, tobacco, marijuana, and other drugs, or a combination of two or more of these substances. More specifically, 1 study focused on tobacco use only (Thomas, McLellan, and Perera, 2015); 2 on illicit drug use only (Faggiano et al., 2014; Ferri et al., 2013); 3 on alcohol and other drug use but not tobacco use (Champion et al., 2013; Tanner-Smith et al., 2015; Thomas, Lorenzetti, and Spragins, 2013); and the remaining 4 on tobacco, alcohol, and other drugs or substance use more broadly (Carney et al., 2016; Hodder et al., 2017; MacArthur et al., 2016; Onrust et al., 2016).

Most programs and interventions in this category were delivered in schools and included universal prevention programs, targeted interventions, or a combination of the two. Additional delivery settings included home or the community (MacArthur et al., 2016), emergency rooms (Tanner-Smith et al., 2015), and mass media campaigns (Ferri et al., 2013). Evidence was not sufficient to suggest that one setting was better than any other, but the overwhelming number of programs provided in schools suggests their utility in reaching a larger population of young people relative to other settings, including those who may not be able to access services outside of school.

Universal programs were delivered in large groups (e.g., whole class), while targeted programs were more often delivered to individuals or in smaller groups. Teachers, peers, and other mentors were the most common facilitators of these programs. In general, adult-led programs were more effective than peer-led programs (Thomas, McLellan, and Perera, 2015), although the latter programs showed some small effects (MacArthur et al., 2016). Some programs also involved parents, who represent an important protective factor for adolescent substance use. For example, Thomas, Lorenzetti, and Spragins (2013) examined the role of mentors and showed that strong family acceptance and community partners helped reduce drug use.

The majority of programs focused exclusively on adolescent populations (range or mean age of 10 to 19), although two of the systematic reviews and meta-analyses also included studies of elementary school–aged children (Faggiano et al., 2014; Hodder et al., 2017; Onrust et al., 2016). In particular, Onrust and colleagues (2016) found significant effects by age, indicating that there are developmental differences in response to program foci and that beginning substance use prevention programs before adolescence can be effective.

Program duration varied considerably, from one brief session to multiple sessions over the course of 2 or more years, and no clear evidence emerged that a specific number of sessions or time spent in a program was more or less beneficial overall. Among targeted programs, two of the studies (Carney et al., 2016; Tanner-Smith et al., 2015) focused on the effects of brief interventions for substance-using adolescents and showed some small effects. Other, more extensive targeted interventions were also effective. For example, Thomas, Lorenzetti, and Spragins (2013) found that frequent meetings helped reduce drug use among substance-using adolescents. Universal prevention programs also ranged in duration, although most of these programs in the reviewed articles were provided over longer periods of time. As mentioned previously, some of these programs began in childhood, highlighting both the developmental differences in program effects and the utility of starting prevention programs early and continuing them through adolescence (Onrust et al., 2016).

Many of the programs were informed by theory, with most using a social competence approach (Botvin, 1983), a social influence approach (Cialdini and Goldstein, 2004), or the transtheoretical model of behavior change (Prochaska and Velicer, 1997). Those using a social competence approach, which aims to reduce or prevent drug use by improving personal and interpersonal skills as well as problem-specific skills, were generally more effective, although the improvement usually was not statistically significant. Those programs based on the social influence model, which attempts to reduce substance use by focusing on social norms and peer influence, were generally less effective and rarely showed statistically significant results. However, programs that used a combination of both the social competence and social influence approaches (e.g., developing interpersonal skills and discussing social norms) were more effective, especially with respect to longer-term outcomes (Faggiano et al., 2014; Thomas, McLellan, and Perera, 2015).

The committee's review of systematic reviews and meta-analyses of programs targeting substance use revealed several promising components, including the utility of school-based programs for universal prevention, programs that begin in childhood, and those that combine social competence and social influence approaches by incorporating skill development with social norm education. Because the studies included were not necessarily designed to identify effective components, our review did not uncover strong evidence in support of specific core components that were consistently effective across multiple studies. Importantly, this lack of evidence may not mean that no such effective components exist. Rather, it represents an opportunity for future research to evaluate the effectiveness of identifiable core components of programs and practices that may be generalizable across different settings and target populations.

Sexual Behavior

Eight different systematic reviews and meta-analyses focused on sexual health. The targeted outcomes varied widely and included both behaviors and health outcomes. Specifically, one article focused on overall sexual health promotion (DeSmet et al., 2015), two focused exclusively on teen pregnancy prevention (Harden et al., 2009; Marseille et al., 2018), one focused exclusively on contraceptive use (Lopez et al., 2016), and one focused on repeat pregnancy prevention (Aslam et al., 2017; Whitaker et al., 2016). The remaining three reviews targeted more than one behavior or outcome: two focused on teen pregnancy and STI prevention (Oringanje et al., 2016; Picot et al., 2012; Shepherd et al., 2010), and one included teen pregnancy and STI prevention as well as sexual risk behaviors (Chin et al., 2012).

Most programs in this category were universal prevention programs, although some were targeted to populations at greater risk for pregnancy and/or STIs, such as teen mothers (Aslam et al., 2017; Whitaker et al., 2016) or specific racial/ethnic groups (Aslam et al., 2017; Whitaker et al., 2016; Marseille et al., 2018; Picot et al., 2012; Shepherd et al., 2010). Some programs were also delivered to separate groups based on biological sex (Harden et al., 2009; Picot et al., 2012; Shepherd et al., 2010).

The most common program settings were schools, followed by community centers. Some programs also occurred at home or in primary care and reproductive health clinics. Programs were most often delivered by teachers and health educators, peers or near-peers, and medical professionals.

The effectiveness of programs delivered in similar settings varied for several reasons. First, not all programs were implemented with fidelity. In school-based settings, for example, implementation was often affected by whether the school was characterized by a supportive school culture, flexible school administration, and enthusiasm and expertise for delivering interactive sessions among teachers and peers (Picot et al., 2012; Shepherd et al., 2010). This finding suggests that creating a supportive and inclusive culture in schools and other program settings can help improve program effectiveness.

Second, not all young people found the programs to be engaging or acceptable. One influential factor in this regard was the qualities of the intervention providers—enthusiasm, credibility, and expertise (in content and in managing groups) (Picot et al., 2012; Shepherd et al., 2010). Other factors were whether the interventions met young people's own needs in relation to sexual health, including sexual feelings, emotions and relationships, the operation of gendered norms, the age-appropriateness of the intervention, and the level of discomfort felt in the classroom setting (Picot et al., 2012; Shepherd et al., 2010). These findings not only provide evidence for creating a supportive and inclusive culture in program settings, but also highlight the importance of including diverse youth and their communities in program development, implementation, and evaluation to ensure that a program meets their needs.

The vast majority of studies reviewed programs for youth ages 10–19, although younger students were sometimes included (Harden et al., 2009; Lopez et al., 2016). The latter were most often early childhood interventions and other youth development programs that provided social support, educational support, and skills training. Many of these early childhood intervention programs also targeted social determinants (e.g., race/ethnicity, socioeconomic status, ability) and structural and systemic issues (e.g., housing, employment opportunities) that affect health, development, and well-being (Harden et al., 2009). Importantly, these early childhood programs appeared to exert a long-term positive influence on the risk of teenage pregnancy, as well as other outcomes associated with social and economic disadvantage, such as unemployment and criminality (Harden et al., 2009). Social and economic disadvantage have not been well addressed in programs and evaluations as determinants of teenage pregnancy (Harden et al., 2009). More research is therefore needed to understand the interdependence of social determinants, structural and systemic issues, behavior, and health outcomes. Furthermore, programs that aim to improve young people's life opportunities, financial circumstances, and future expectations represent an important avenue for future work.

The frequency and duration of the programs studied varied significantly, from brief, single sessions to multiple sessions over a number of years. Comparisons by program duration showed that those provided over a longer period were more effective than those delivered as single sessions, a finding attributed to the fact that such programs give participants more opportunities to practice the skills they have learned (Picot et al., 2012; Shepherd et al., 2010).

As was found for the substance use studies, the sexual health studies included in the committee's review generally were not designed to identify program components that were more effective than others. However, the body of evidence presented in these reviews highlights the potential effectiveness and generalizability of particular approaches. First, creating a supportive and inclusive culture in program settings and including diverse youth and their communities in program development, implementation, and evaluation efforts can ensure that such programs meet the needs of the youth they target. This is a prevalent theme not only in the literature, but also in the experiences of current Teen Pregnancy Prevention (TPP) program Tier 1B implementation grantees (Baltimore City Health Department, 2019; Mary Black Foundation, 2019; Methodist Le Bonheur Community Outreach, 2019; Morehouse School of Medicine, 2019; San Diego Youth Services, 2019; The Center for Black Women's Wellness Inc., 2019).

Second, traditional approaches to reducing teenage pregnancy rates, such as inclusive sex education and better sexual health services, can be complemented, but not replaced, by positive youth development programs. The latter programs use behavioral theory–based approaches to increase adolescents' knowledge; influence their attitudes and beliefs; create supportive norms; and build relevant communication, decision-making, and practical skills that help build self-efficacy. These programs are associated with prevention and decreased risk of pregnancy, HIV infection, and STIs (Chin et al., 2012; DeSmet et al., 2015; Lopez et al., 2016; Marseille et al., 2018). Future research is needed to evaluate the core components of these programs that can be effective across multiple behaviors and outcomes.

Emotional Health

Six of the systematic reviews and meta-analyses focused on emotional health (Calear and Christensen, 2010; Clarke, Kuosmanen, and Barry, 2015; Corrieri et al., 2014; Das et al., 2016; Dray et al., 2017; van Genugten et al., 2017). All six addressed specific types of internalizing symptoms or behaviors (e.g., depression or anxiety symptoms, low self-esteem, stress), while three also included externalizing symptoms or behaviors (e.g., conduct problems, violence) (Das et al., 2016; Dray et al., 2017; van Genugten et al., 2017).[7]

Four of the systematic reviews and meta-analyses included programs delivered only in school settings (Calear and Christensen, 2010; Corrieri et al., 2014; Dray et al., 2017; van Genugten et al., 2017). The other two included programs provided in schools and at least one other setting, including primary care clinics (Das et al., 2016) or through digital platforms (Clarke, Kuosmanen, and Barry, 2015). All six systematic reviews and meta-analyses included programs focused on universal prevention of emotional health problems, while most also included programs targeted to adolescents considered at risk based on family history or symptoms (Calear and Christensen, 2010; Clarke, Kuosmanen, and Barry, 2015;

---

[7]Articles that focused only on samples of adolescents with diagnosed mental health disorders (e.g., depression, anxiety, attention deficit-hyperactivity disorder) were excluded because these represent chronic medical conditions.

Corrieri et al., 2014; Das et al., 2016; van Genugten et al., 2017). The fact that the majority of these programs occurred, at least in part, in schools again suggests the usefulness of schools in addressing adolescent health and well-being.

Most universal programs were administered in group settings, except for those in the Clarke, Kuosmanen, and Barry (2015) study, which were all self-administered through digital media platforms. Targeted programs were delivered both individually and in group settings. Programs were most often provided by teachers, trained external facilitators (e.g., mental health providers, researchers, health professionals), or some combination of the two. Although digital e-health interventions showed some promise for improving emotional health, participant retention was lower in programs delivered exclusively through digital media compared with those that also included an in-person component, indicating the value of in-person time for these types of programs (Clarke, Kuosmanen, and Barry, 2015; Das et al., 2016).

In general, emotional health programs involved more frequent and more consistent sessions relative to the substance use and sexual health programs included in our review. The majority of programs included multiple sessions, ranging from two total meetings to daily sessions over the course of 36 weeks.

The average age of program recipients for each study was 10–19, although children as young as 5 and late adolescents as old as 25 were included in some of the systematic reviews and meta-analyses. Four of the studies also examined programs involving parents as a complement to school-based programs (Calear and Christensen, 2010; Corrieri et al., 2014; Das et al., 2016; Dray et al., 2017).

Overall, programs informed by cognitive-behavioral therapy (CBT) techniques were shown to be effective in improving emotional health across all the systematic reviews and meta-analyses. The goal of CBT is to change the automatic negative thoughts that contribute to emotional distress and related behavior problems, and such therapies have strong evidence of effectiveness for a variety of internalizing and externalizing problems across ages and demographic subgroups (Hofmann et al., 2012). Among the studies included in our review, those that used CBT techniques to promote resilience, self-regulation, and coping skills were most consistently associated with decreased internalizing and externalizing symptoms and improved emotional well-being (Calear and Christensen, 2010; Clarke, Kuosmanen, and Barry, 2015; Corrieri et al., 2014; Das et al., 2016; Dray et al., 2017; van Genugten et al., 2017).

As with the studies in the physical health domain, none of those identified in the emotional health domain were specifically designed to identify core components. This made it difficult for the committee to definitively isolate those program elements that are most effective in promoting emotional health. However, several key characteristics of programs show great promise in addressing internalizing and/or externalizing symptoms or behaviors related to emotional health. In general, programs that were provided universally, in school, with some in-person meeting, with multiple sessions over a greater number of weeks, and with the incorporation of CBT techniques showed some effectiveness for promoting emotional health among adolescents.

These results reflect those of other research on core components of mental health programs for youth. While our review did not include studies of adolescents with diagnosed mental health conditions, much of the seminal work on core components comes from this field. For example, core components research has shown that exposure to a fear or stressor may be the most important component of CBT for anxiety and traumatic stress (Seligman and Ollendick, 2011). Studies using similar approaches to identify the core components of prevention programs for emotional health will therefore be an important area for future research.

Social Health

No studies in our review focused exclusively on social health. This is likely because social health is often integrated into programs focused on social-emotional learning and positive youth development. Studies that include social health among the domains covered are discussed in greater detail in the section below on multiple optimal health domains.

Spiritual Health

As with social health, no studies in our review focused exclusively on spiritual health. However, a number of studies included outcomes related to spiritual health in combination with other areas of optimal health. These are described in the section on multiple optimal health domains as well.

Intellectual Health

Only one study in our review exclusively examined intellectual health outcomes (Hahn et al., 2015; Wilson et al., 2011). Unlike the studies in the other domains, this comprehensive meta-analysis was designed specifically to identify core components and thus to provide evidence for effective components of programs targeting intellectual health outcomes.

The authors of this study conducted a meta-analysis of programs and interventions aimed at increasing high school participation rates. They included 152 studies in their meta-analysis,[8] and the outcomes of interest included school enrollment, school dropout, and completion of a high school degree or the General Education Development (GED) tests. Programs included in the review fell into the following categories: attendance monitoring, multiservice packages, alternative schools, supplemental academic training, case management, school/class restructuring, skills training/CBT, college preparation, mentoring/counseling, vocational training, community service, and others. The vast majority of programs took place in schools, with others being delivered in community settings or in a combination of school and community settings. Most programs entailed daily contact with participants, and program duration averaged about two school years. The average age of participants was 15, although some programs targeted elementary school–aged children.

Broadly, this meta-analysis found that programs taking place in schools and those delivered in multiple settings (including schools) were more effective than those offered in community settings. It also found that all program types except those designated as "other" showed significant effectiveness in decreasing school dropout rates among program participants compared with the average dropout rate. Furthermore, while most categories of programs were equally effective, programs focused on attendance monitoring were significantly less successful than programs in most of the other categories.

It is significant that almost half of the studies in this review reported issues with program implementation, including structural issues (e.g., access to resources), staffing issues, funding issues, and difficulties obtaining administrator buy-in. This suggests that having supportive school environments and improved access to resources may help promote positive program effects. In addition, given the economic and health benefits of education, the provision of these additional services to socially disadvantaged youth can help improve their life opportunities and promote equity. Therefore, actions to create supportive school culture and promote equitable access to resources can have major impacts on adolescents' overall health and well-being.

Multiple Optimal Health Domains

Given the interrelatedness of the dimensions of optimal health, it is not surprising that six of the systematic reviews and meta-analyses considered the effects of programs on outcomes in multiple optimal health domains

---

[8]An additional 15 programs for teen mothers were included in the review but were analyzed separately given these participants' specialized needs. Our summary is based on the 152 studies that were offered to broader populations of youth.

(Ciocanel et al., 2017; Durlak et al., 2011; Durlak, Weissberg, and Pachan, 2010; Klingbeil et al., 2017; MacArthur et al., 2018; Taylor et al., 2017). The behaviors and outcomes targeted in these reviews included substance use, pregnancy, sexual behavior, positive social behavior, academic performance, emotional distress, mindfulness, and self-regulation skills, among others. Despite this broad scope of outcomes, this part of the committee's review ultimately encompasses the most consequential components of optimal health. Instead of focusing on a narrowly targeted behavior, the programs reviewed in this section attempted to teach skills that, if learned successfully, underlie and impact health in multiple domains and across the life course.

Most of the programs reviewed in these articles used a social-emotional learning or positive youth development framework. Both of these frameworks posit that supporting social and emotional skills and positive attitudes helps youth develop social and emotional assets that have positive effects on well-being and are protective against negative outcomes (Ciocanel et al., 2017; Durlak et al., 2011; Durlak, Weissberg, and Pachan, 2010; Taylor et al., 2017).

Klingbeil and colleagues (2017) studied mindfulness-based interventions, which similarly sought to provide youth with self-regulation and acceptance skills to improve physical, emotional, social, spiritual, and intellectual health outcomes. These skills are challenging to target through interventions, perhaps because they are difficult to measure and test. That said, these are skills that are required for some of the most important developmental tasks of adolescence. Also, many programs included in this study did show significant measurable effects on the outcomes of interest, effects that were maintained for as long as 18 months or more.

The programs addressed in these articles were most often delivered in schools or multiple locations that included schools (Dray et al., 2017; Durlak et al., 2011; MacArthur et al., 2018; Taylor et al., 2017) or in after school and community-based settings (Ciocanel et al., 2017; Durlak, Weissberg, and Pachan, 2010). Across multiple articles in our review, school-based programs that were provided universally to all students showed the strongest evidence of effectiveness (Durlak et al., 2011; MacArthur et al., 2018). This finding provides further support for the findings described earlier, suggesting that schools are particularly well suited for providing programs that have positive effects on multiple optimal health-related outcomes.

Participants in these programs were ages 5–18. Although the average age of participants was 10–19, these programs were more likely to include younger children relative to those described in previous subsections. Notably, there were reported differences in program effects by age. In particular, the Taylor et al. (2017) study found that programs for younger children (ages 5–10) had significantly greater effects on measured outcomes compared with those for early adolescents (ages 11–13). However, effects did not differ between mid- to late adolescents (ages 14–18) and the younger age groups. Similarly, Dray and colleagues (2017) found that for younger children, resilience-focused programs were more effective in decreasing anxiety symptoms and emotional distress, whereas for adolescents, these programs were more effective in decreasing internalizing problems. Evidence from these studies provides further support for the value of starting programs early in the life course and for providing such programs at multiple stages of development to capitalize on the critical developmental windows between early childhood and young adulthood.

Another important finding from Taylor et al. (2017) and other studies was that there were few to no differences in program effects by demographic characteristics. More specifically, the positive effects of social-emotional learning and positive youth development programs were statistically equivalent for students of different racial/ethnic backgrounds and socioeconomic levels. Such findings indicate the value of these programs in achieving equitable, positive outcomes for *all* youth, regardless of background.

Program design and implementation were also critical components for program success. Programs that could be described by the SAFE acronym were most successful in producing positive effects on social, emotional, and intellectual health outcomes (Durlak et al., 2011; Durlak, Weissberg, and Pachan, 2010; Taylor et al., 2017). The SAFE acronym, which represents the design and implementation components that have been shown to be effective in producing positive outcomes, refers to programs that are (1) *sequenced* and have step-by-step training for facilitators, (2) include aspects of *active* learning, (3) have *focused* attention and adequate time devoted to skills training, and (4) have *explicit* definitions of program goals. Programs with the SAFE designation were consistently found to be more effective than those that did not have these characteristics, highlighting the importance of program design and fidelity in prevention and intervention programs.

Overall, the committee's examination of this literature aligns with the five core social-emotional learning competencies developed by the Collaborative for Academic, Social, and Emotional Learning (CASEL) (2019). These competencies represent the foundational skills that programs might seek to achieve to promote healthy behaviors and outcomes for youth:

- *Self-awareness*: "The ability to accurately recognize one's own emotions, thoughts, and values and how they influence behavior. The ability to accurately assess one's strengths and limitations, with a well-grounded sense of confidence, optimism, and a 'growth mindset.'" (para. 2)

- *Self-management*: "The ability to successfully regulate one's emotions, thoughts, and behaviors in different situations—effectively managing stress, controlling impulses, and motivating oneself. The ability to set and work toward personal and academic goals." (para. 3)
- *Social awareness*: "The ability to take the perspective of and empathize with others, including those from diverse backgrounds and cultures. The ability to understand social and ethical norms for behavior and to recognize family, school, and community resources and supports." (para. 4)
- *Relationship skills*: "The ability to establish and maintain healthy and rewarding relationships with diverse individuals and groups. The ability to communicate clearly, listen well, cooperate with others, resist inappropriate social pressure, negotiate conflict constructively, and seek and offer help when needed." (para. 5)
- *Responsible decision making*: "The ability to make constructive choices about personal behavior and social interactions based on ethical standards, safety concerns, and social norms. The realistic evaluation of consequences of various actions, and a consideration of the well-being of oneself and others." (para. 6)

Summary

In summary, the committee's ability to identify specific and discrete core program components was limited by the scope of the systematic reviews and meta-analyses currently available in the literature. Although we did not find consistent evidence of effectiveness for particular core components across all of the studies reviewed, several of the evaluated programs show promise across multiple domains of optimal health (see Box 4-1). In particular, social-emotional learning and positive youth development programs offer great potential benefit, as they are aimed at equipping children and adolescents with the foundational skills they need to engage in impulse control and self-regulation, skills that ultimately help them make healthy decisions in a variety of situations.

Importantly, while few of the papers in our review included digital e-health interventions, we recognize that this is more likely due to the age of the included studies rather than a representation of their utility. Since smartphones and computers have become nearly ubiquitous among adolescents today compared with even 5 years ago (Anderson and Jiang, 2018) (see Chapter 2), further investigation of the effectiveness of digitally delivered interventions among more contemporary cohorts of youth is needed.

BOX 4-1
Promising Components Identified in the Systematic Review,
by Optimal Health Domain

Physical Health
Substance use:
- Universal programs
- Being school based
- Beginning in childhood
- Combining social competence and social influence approaches

Sexual behavior:
- Beginning in childhood
- Creating a supportive and inclusive culture in program settings
- Including diverse youth and their communities in program development, implementation, and evaluation efforts
- Promoting skills based on social-emotional learning and positive youth development as a complement to inclusive sex education and sexual health services

Emotional Health
- Universal programs
- Being school based
- Including in-person meetings
- Multiple sessions over longer periods of time
- Incorporating cognitive-behavioral therapy techniques

Intellectual Health
- Providing programs in schools or a combination of schools and other settings
- Promoting supportive school culture and access to resources

Multiple Optimal Health Domains
- Promoting competencies based on social-emotional learning and positive youth development
- Starting interventions in childhood
- Being sequenced, active, focused, and explicit

RESULTS OF CORE COMPONENTS PAPER REVIEW

In addition to the systematic review of systematic reviews and meta-analyses reported above, the committee identified a selected group of papers that were clearly focused on core components of effective practice for improving outcomes in each of the optimal health domains. These papers used methodologies of systematic reviews or meta-analyses (Boustani et al., 2015) or were reviews of reviews (Peters et al., 2009). We used the results of our review of these papers to supplement the findings obtained from our systematic review and to ensure that the most current research on core components would be explored and considered.

While a number of papers made reference to core components or elements, these articles were often focused on a specific program instead of considering the shared components of multiple programs. Findings from the four articles that met the final criteria for our core components review are summarized below (Boustani et al., 2015; Lawson et al., 2019; Peters et al., 2009; Tolan et al., 2016).

Boustani et al. (2015)

Boustani and colleagues (2015) identified common elements that exist across evidence-based prevention programs for multiple health behaviors and outcomes, including substance use, life skills, sexual health, violence, and depression/anxiety. To this end, they used a distillation and matching approach, which entails systematically reviewing EBPs to aggregate the core components that are most common to these programs and are thus likely to be the most effective (Chorpita et al., 2005). As the authors state:

> The current findings lend initial support for this method of knowledge aggregation to identify a core set of skills designed to reduce common pathways to risk behaviors such as conduct problems and substance use— and to prepare youth for healthy trajectories characterized by successful relationships, prosocial behaviors, sexual health, and positive adjustment (Boustani et al., 2015, p. 215).

Across prevention programs for all outcomes, Boustani and colleagues (2015) found that problem solving was the most common practice component, followed by communication skills, assertiveness training, and insight building. The most common instructional components were psychoeducation, modeling, and role play (see Figure 4-7).

Although their review identified common components of these programs, the authors provide no statistical evidence that any of these components were more or less effective than others. This represents an important next step for future research.

Lawson et al. (2019)

CASEL is a compilation of evidence-based programs meant to facilitate social-emotional learning. While a number of such programs have been found to be successful, Lawson and colleagues (2019) suggest that a core set of components appears across programs. They first selected programs from the CASEL database that met the following criteria:

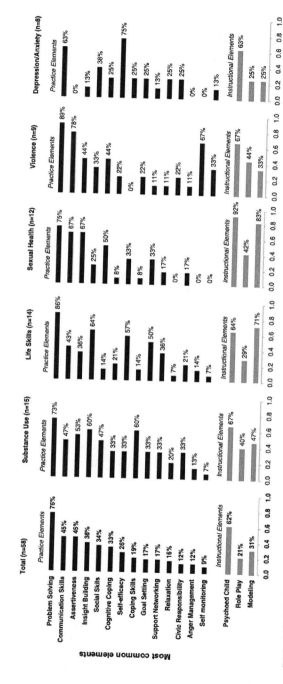

FIGURE 4-7 Common components of adolescent prevention programs.

SOURCE: Boustani et al. (2015). Republished with permission of Taylor & Francis, Ltd. Permission conveyed through Copyright Clearance Center, Inc.

- targets all five areas of CASEL competence (self-awareness, self-management, social awareness, relationship skills, and responsible decision making);
- provides opportunities to practice;
- offers multiyear programming;
- offers training and other implementation support;
- has at least one evaluation study that included a comparison group and pre–post measures; and
- documents a positive impact on one of the four outcome domains (academics, conduct problems, emotional distress, prosocial behavior).

Next, the authors coded the components present in each of the 14 programs included in their final sample. The most common components were social skills (100% of programs), identifying others' feelings (100% of programs), behavioral coping skills/relaxation (92.9% of programs), and identifying one's own feelings (87.7% of programs). The least commonly addressed components were mindfulness (20% of programs), valuing diversity (63.6% of programs), cognitive coping/self-talk (75% of programs), and goal setting and planning (75% of programs).

Importantly, this review identified components that were present or absent in programs that had been determined to be efficacious, rather than testing the effectiveness of each component on its own. Testing for the effectiveness of each of these core components of social-emotional learning programs thus represents an important area for future research.

Tolan et al. (2016)

Tolan and colleagues (2016) took a broad and integrative approach to understanding a range of factors that might influence positive youth development. They compared four interrelated frameworks: social competence (SC) (Waters and Sroufe, 1983), social-emotional learning (SEL) (Elias, Zins, and Weissberg, 1997), positive youth development (PYD) (Lerner et al., 2002), and positive psychology (PPsy) (Seligman and Csikszentmihalyi, 2014). A major objective of the review was to identify core components across orientations, with a focus on developing a "unified framework to guide interventions" (Tolan et al., 2016, p. 215). The authors concluded that four core components are consistent across the models they reviewed and that these components facilitate positive outcomes: self-control, positive self-orientation, engagement with others, and societal bonding/moral ethical standards. Although each framework defines and measures these constructs slightly differently (see Table 4-2), they are nevertheless consistent themes that could serve as intervention targets to promote optimal

TABLE 4-2 Common Construct Threads and Potential Alignment Across the Four Frameworks

Overarching constructs	SC	SEL	PYD	PPsy
Self-control	Self-control	Self-management	Character Competence	Accomplishment/ Achievement
Positive self-orientation	Positive sense of self	Self-awareness	Confidence	Positive emotions
Engagement with others	Prosocial connectedness	Relationship skills Social awareness	Connection	Engagement & positive relationships
Societal bonding/ Moral ethical standards	Moral system of belief & decision-making skills	Responsible decision making	Caring/ Compassion	Meaning

SOURCE: Tolan et al. (2016). Republished with permission of Springer Nature. Permission conveyed through Copyright Clearance Center, Inc.

health. Again, isolating and measuring the effects of these common components will be an important consideration for future research.

Peters et al. (2009)

As noted above in the discussion of the committee's systematic review, schools are a common setting for many behavioral interventions; however, many school health education programs focus on a single behavioral domain. In contrast, integrative, multicomponent programs that address multiple behaviors may be more efficient. The review by Peters and colleagues (2009) suggests that this efficiency is enhanced if the elements of change are similar across all of the targeted behaviors and outcomes.

These authors conducted a systematic review of the effectiveness of school-based health promotion programs targeting substance use, sexual behavior, and nutrition.[9] The 55 reviews included in their analysis yielded five core components deemed effective across all three targeted behaviors: being theory-based; addressing social influences (especially social norms); addressing cognitive-behavioral skills; including the training of facilitators; and consisting of multiple components. "Tentative" evidence also suggested

---

[9]This paper indicates positive, negative, or no statistically significant effect of each program component, but does not report effect sizes. This reporting method makes it more difficult to compare the magnitudes of these effects.

positive effects of parent involvement and a greater number of sessions. In contrast, a knowledge-only approach was not effective in any of the above three domains, although the strength of evidence varied. All of these findings complement those identified in our systematic review.

Some components were more effective than others for certain groups of outcomes. In the domains of sexuality and nutrition programs, programs with a specific behavioral focus were more effective than those that addressed general issues (e.g., condom use vs. general sexuality). In addition, evidence indicated that addressing behavioral determinants and tailoring to cognitive ability or age were effective in these two domains. Strong and moderate reviews of sexuality and substance use programs indicated that tailoring interventions to the culture of the target group was also effective.

Sexuality and substance use programs both addressed abstinence goals, and strong reviews in both domains indicated their ineffectiveness and even their negative effects in some cases. Specifically, the authors state that "not one sexuality review stated positive conclusions about the effectiveness of abstinence-only programs, which portray abstinence from sex as the only or very best prevention option and usually do not discuss contraception," and further state that one sexuality review "even reported negative effects." For substance use, the authors state that "harm reduction or prevention of abuse may be more effective than a goal of abstinence or delayed use, at least for youth who already use."

Summary

In summary, the additional papers the committee reviewed identify common components of effective programs, although statistical evidence is rarely provided to suggest that any of the components is more or less effective than others (see Box 4-2). Future work is needed in this area to provide a more complete understanding of the ways in which these components compare directly with one another, as well as the ways in which their efficacy may vary by particular demographic groups.

CONCLUSIONS

With respect to core components of programs that are effective in promoting positive adolescent health behaviors and outcomes, the committee drew the following conclusions.

CONCLUSION 4-1: Most current research is not designed to identify which components of adolescent risk behavior programs or interventions are more effective than others.

BOX 4-2
Common Components Identified in the
Supplemental Paper Review

Most Common Components in Effective Programs
(evidence of effectiveness of specific components not provided)

Boustani et al. (2015)
Practice components:
- Problem solving
- Communication skills
- Assertiveness training
- Insight building

Instructional components:
- Psychoeducation
- Modeling
- Role play

Lawson et al. (2019)
- Social skills
- Identifying others' feelings
- Behavioral coping skills/relaxation
- Identifying one's own feelings

Tolan et al. (2016)
- Self-control
- Positive self-orientation
- Engagement with others
- Societal bonding/moral ethical standards

Components of Programs with Evidence of Effectiveness
(magnitude of effects not reported)

Peters et al. (2009)
All programs:
- Being theory-based
- Addressing social influences (especially social norms)
- Cognitive-behavioral skills
- Training facilitators
- Consisting of multiple components

Substance use and sexual behavior programs:
- Harm reduction or prevention rather than abstinence-only or delayed use

---

CONCLUSION 4-2: More research is needed to determine how, when, and for whom the common components of programs are effective in promoting positive adolescent health behaviors and outcomes.

CONCLUSION 4-3: Programs that are sequenced, include an active learning technique, have focused time devoted to skills training, and have explicit program goals are more effective than those that lack these characteristics.

CONCLUSION 4-4: Programs that incorporate approaches based on behavioral theory, social-emotional learning, and positive youth development are more successful in promoting positive adolescent health behaviors and outcomes across multiple optimal health domains relative to those that do not use these approaches to inform programmatic efforts.

CONCLUSION 4-5: Multicomponent, multisession programs focused on social-emotional learning and positive youth development that emphasize knowledge, attitudes, and skills are more successful in supporting healthy adolescent development than programs focused on individual risk behaviors.

CONCLUSION 4-6: Efforts to assist adolescents in making healthy decisions related to risk-taking behaviors—including alcohol and tobacco use and sexual activity, among others—need to begin in early childhood and continue through adolescence.

CONCLUSION 4-7: Programs that target social determinants of health and well-being can have widespread, positive effects on multiple behaviors and outcomes.

CONCLUSION 4-8: Having supportive environments and improved access to resources can lead to greater positive program effects.

CONCLUSION 4-9: Program development, implementation, and evaluation efforts would benefit from including youth of diverse ages, racial/ethnic backgrounds, socioeconomic status, rurality/urbanity, sexual orientations, sexes/genders, and disability/ability status.

The next and final chapter of this report provides the committee's recommendations—based on the conclusions presented in Chapters 2 through 4—for research and the Office of the Assistant Secretary for Health's programs and policies.

REFERENCES

Anderson, M., and Jiang, J. (2018). *Teens, Social Media & Technology 2018*. Washington, DC: Pew Research Center.

Aslam, R.W., Hendry, M., Booth, A., Carter, B., Charles, J.M., Craine, N., Edwards, R.T., Noyes, J., Ntambwe, L.I., Pasterfield, D., Rycroft-Malone, J., Williams, N., and Whitaker, R. (2017). Intervention now to eliminate repeat unintended pregnancy in teenagers (INTERUPT): A systematic review of intervention effectiveness and cost-effectiveness, and qualitative and realist synthesis of implementation factors and user engagement. *BMC Medicine, 15*(1), 155.

Baltimore City Health Department. (2019). TPP Grantee Memo: Baltimore City Health Department U Choose program. Memo to the Committee on Applying Lessons of Optimal Adolescent Health to Improve Behavioral Outcomes for Youth. Baltimore City, MD: Baltimore City Health Department.

Barth, R.P., and Liggett-Creel, K. (2014). Common components of parenting programs for children birth to eight years of age involved with child welfare services. *Children and Youth Services Review, 40*, 6–12.

Blase, K., and Fixsen, D. (2013). *Core Intervention Components: Identifying and Operationalizing What Makes Programs Work. ASPE Research Brief.* U.S. Department of Health and Human Services. Available: https://aspe.hhs.gov/report/core-intervention-components-identifying-and-operationalizing-what-makes-programs-work.

Botvin, G.J. (1983). Prevention of adolescent substance abuse through the development of personal and social competence. *Preventing Adolescent Drug Abuse: Intervention Strategies*, 115–140.

Boustani, M.M., Frazier, S.L., Becker, K.D., Bechor, M., Dinizulu, S.M., Hedemann, E.R., Ogle, R.R., and Pasalich, D.S. (2015). Common elements of adolescent prevention programs: Minimizing burden while maximizing reach. *Administration and Policy in Mental Health and Mental Health Services Research, 42*(2), 209–219.

Calear, A.L., and Christensen, H. (2010). Systematic review of school-based prevention and early intervention programs for depression. *Journal of Adolescence, 33*(3), 429–438.

Carney, T., Myers, B.J., Louw, J., and Okwundu, C.I. (2016). Brief school-based interventions and behavioural outcomes for substance-using adolescents. *Cochrane Database of Systematic Reviews*(1), Cd008969.

Centers for Disease Control and Prevention (CDC). (2017). *Picture of America: Prevention.* Atlanta, GA: Author.

Champion, K.E., Newton, N.C., Barrett, E.L., and Teesson, M. (2013). A systematic review of school-based alcohol and other drug prevention programs facilitated by computers or the internet. *Drug and Alcohol Review, 32*(2), 115–123.

Chin, H.B., Sipe, T.A., Elder, R., Mercer, S.L., Chattopadhyay, S.K., Jacob, V., Wethington, H.R., Kirby, D., Elliston, D.B., Griffith, M., Chuke, S.O., Briss, S.C., Ericksen, I., Galbraith, J.S., Herbst, J.H., Johnson, R.L., Kraft, J.M., Noar, S.M., Romero, L.M., and Santelli, J. (2012). The effectiveness of group-based comprehensive risk-reduction and abstinence education interventions to prevent or reduce the risk of adolescent pregnancy, human immunodeficiency virus, and sexually transmitted infections: Two systematic reviews for the Guide to Community Preventive Services. *American Journal of Preventive Medicine, 42*(3), 272–294.

Chorpita, B.F., and Daleiden, E.L. (2009). Mapping evidence-based treatments for children and adolescents: Application of the distillation and matching model to 615 treatments from 322 randomized trials. *Journal of Consulting and Clinical Psychology, 77*(3), 566–579.

Chorpita, B.F., Delaiden, E.L., and Weisz, J.R. (2005). Identifying and selecting the common elements of evidence based interventions: A distillation and matching model. *Mental Health Services Research, 7*, 5–20.

Cialdini, R.B., and Goldstein, N.J. (2004). Social influence: Compliance and conformity. *Annual Review of Psychology, 55*, 591–621.

Ciocanel, O., Power, K., Eriksen, A., and Gillings, K. (2017). Effectiveness of positive youth development interventions: A meta-analysis of randomized controlled trials. *Journal of Youth and Adolescence, 46*(3), 483–504.

Clarke, A.M., Kuosmanen, T., and Barry, M.M. (2015). A systematic review of online youth mental health promotion and prevention interventions. *Journal of Youth and Adolescence, 44*(1), 90–113.

Collaborative for Academic, Social, and Emotional Learning. (2019). *Core SEL Competencies.* Available: https://casel.org/core-competencies.

Corrieri, S., Heider, D., Conrad, I., Blume, A., Konig, H-H., and Riedel-Heller, S.G. (2014). School-based prevention programs for depression and anxiety in adolescence: A systematic review. *Health Promotion International, 29*(3), 427–441.

Das, J.K., Salam, R.A., Lassi, Z.S., Khan, M.N., Mahmood, W., Patel, V., and Bhutta, Z.A. (2016). Interventions for adolescent mental health: An overview of systematic reviews. *Journal of Adolescent Health, 59*(4S), S49–S60.

David P. Weikart Center for Youth Program Quality. (2019). *Youth Program Quality Assessment® and School-Age Program Quality Assessment.* Available: http://cypq.org/assessment.

DeSmet, A., Shegog, R., Van Ryckeghem, D., Crombez, G., and De Bourdeaudhuij, I. (2015). A systematic review and meta-analysis of interventions for sexual health promotion involving serious digital games. *Games and Health Journal, 4*(2), 78–90.

Dray, J., Bowman, J., Campbell, E., Freund, M., Wolfenden, L., Hodder, R.K., McElwaine, K., Tremain, D., Bartlem, K., Bailey, J., Small, T., Palazzi, K., Oldmeadow, C., and Wiggers, J. (2017). Systematic review of universal resilience-focused interventions targeting child and adolescent mental health in the school setting. *Journal of the American Academy of Child & Adolescent Psychiatry, 56*(10), 813–824.

Durlak, J.A., Weissberg, R.P., Dymnicki, A.B., Taylor, R.D., and Schellinger, K.B. (2011). The impact of enhancing students' social and emotional learning: A meta-analysis of school-based universal interventions. *Child Development, 82*(1), 405–432.

Durlak, J.A., Weissberg, R.P., and Pachan, M. (2010). A meta-analysis of after-school programs that seek to promote personal and social skills in children and adolescents. *American Journal of Community Psychology, 45*(3–4), 294–309.

Elias, M.J., Zins, J.E., and Weissberg, R.P. (1997). *Promoting Social and Emotional Learning: Guidelines for Educators.* Alexandria, VA: Association for Supervision and Curriculum Development.

Embry, D.D., and Biglan, A. (2008). Evidence-based kernels: Fundamental units of behavioral influence. *Clinical Child and Family Psychology Review, 11*(3), 75–113.

Faggiano, F., Minozzi, S., Versino, E., and Buscemi, D. (2014). Universal school-based prevention for illicit drug use. *Cochrane Database of Systematic Reviews*(12), Cd003020.

Ferri, M., Allara, E., Bo, A., Gasparrini, A., and Faggiano, F. (2013). Media campaigns for the prevention of illicit drug use in young people. *Cochrane Database of Systematic Reviews*(6), Cd009287.

Gordon, R.S. (1983). An operational classification of disease prevention. *Public Health Reports, 98*(2), 107.

Hahn, R.A., Knopf, J.A., Wilson, S.J., Truman, B.I., Milstein, B., Johnson, R.L., Fielding, J.E., Muntaner, C.J.M., Jones, C.P., Fullilove, M.T., Moss, R.D., Ueffing, E., and Hunt, P.C. (2015). Programs to increase high school completion: A Community Guide systematic health equity review. *American Journal of Preventive Medicine, 48*(5), 599–608.

Harden, A., Brunton, G., Fletcher, A., and Oakley, A. (2009). Teenage pregnancy and social disadvantage: Systematic review integrating controlled trials and qualitative studies. *British Medical Journal, 339*, b4254.

Hodder, R.K., Freund, M., Wolfenden, L., Bowman, J., Nepal, S., Dray, J., Kingsland, M., Yoong, S.L., and Wiggers, J. (2017). Systematic review of universal school-based 'resilience' interventions targeting adolescent tobacco, alcohol or illicit substance use: A meta-analysis. *Preventive Medicine, 100*, 248–268.

Hofmann, S.G., Asnaani, A., Vonk, I.J.J., Sawyer, A.T., and Fang, A. (2012). The efficacy of cognitive behavioral therapy: A review of meta-analyses. *Cognitive Therapy and Research, 36*(5), 427–440.

Hogue, A., Bobek, M., Dauber, S., Henderson, C.E., McLeod, B.D., and Southam-Gerow, M.A. (2017). Distilling the core elements of family therapy for adolescent substance use: Conceptual and empirical solutions. *Journal of Child & Adolescent Substance Abuse, 26*(6), 437–453.

Institute of Medicine. (1994). *Reducing Risks for Mental Disorders: Frontiers for Preventive Intervention Research*. Washington, DC: The National Academies Press.

Katz, D.L., and Ali, A. (2009). *Preventive Medicine, Integrative Medicine, and the Health of the Public*. Washington, DC: Institute of Medicine.

Klingbeil, D.A., Renshaw, T.L., Willenbrink, J.B., Copek, R.A., Chan, K.T., Haddock, A., Yassine, J., and Clifton, J. (2017). Mindfulness-based interventions with youth: A comprehensive meta-analysis of group-design studies. *Journal of School Psychology, 63*, 77–103.

Lawson, G.M., McKenzie, M.E., Becker, K.D., Selby, L., and Hoover, S.A. (2019). The core components of evidence-based social emotional learning programs. *Prevention Science, 20*(4), 457–467.

Lerner, R.M., Brentano, C., Dowling, E.M., and Anderson, P.M. (2002). Positive youth development: Thriving as the basis of personhood and civil society. *New Directions for Youth Development, 2002*(95), 11–34.

Lipsey, M.W. (2018). Effective use of the large body of research on the effectiveness of programs for juvenile offenders and the failure of the model programs approach. *Criminology & Public Policy, 17*(1), 189–198.

Lopez, L.M., Bernholc, A., Chen, M., and Tolley, E.E. (2016). School-based interventions for improving contraceptive use in adolescents. *Cochrane Database of Systematic Reviews*(6), Cd012249.

MacArthur, G., Caldwell, D.M., Redmore, J., Watkins, S.H., Kipping, R., White, J., Chittleborough, C., Langford, R., Er, V., Lingam, R., Pasch, K., Gunnell, D., Hickman, M., and Campbell, R. (2018). Individual-, family-, and school-level interventions targeting multiple risk behaviours in young people. *Cochrane Database of Systematic Reviews*(10).

MacArthur, G.J., Harrison, S., Caldwell, D.M., Hickman, M., and Campbell, R. (2016). Peer-led interventions to prevent tobacco, alcohol and/or drug use among young people aged 11–21 years: A systematic review and meta-analysis. *Addiction, 111*(3), 391–407.

Marseille, E., Mirzazadeh, A., Biggs, M.A., Miller, A.P., Horvath, H., Lightfoot, M., Malekinejad, M., and Kahn, J.G. (2018). Effectiveness of school-based teen pregnancy prevention programs in the USA: A systematic review and meta-analysis. *Prevention Science, 19*(4), 468–489.

Mary Black Foundation. (2019). TPP grantee memo: Mary Black Foundation. *Memo to the Committee on Applying Lessons of Optimal Adolescent Health to Improve Behavioral Outcomes for Youth*. Spartanburg, SC: Mary Black Foundation.

Methodist Le Bonheur Community Outreach. (2019). TPP grantee memo: Methodist Le Bonheur Community Outreach. *Memo to the Committee on Applying Lessons of Optimal Adolescent Health to Improve Behavioral Outcomes for Youth*. Memphis, TN: Methodist Le Bonheur Community Outreach.

Moher, D., Liberati, A., Tetzlaff, J., and Altman, D.G. (2009). Preferred reporting items for systematic reviews and meta-analyses: The PRISMA statement. *Annals of Internal Medicine, 151*(4), 264–269.

Morehouse School of Medicine. (2019). *TPP Grantee Memo: Morehouse School of Medicine's Carrera Program*. Memo to the Committee on Applying Lessons of Optimal Adolescent Health to Improve Behavioral Outcomes for Youth. Atlanta, GA: Morehouse School of Medicine.

National Academies of Sciences, Engineering, and Medicine (NASEM). (2019). *Applying Lessons of Optimal Adolescent Health to Improve Behavioral Outcomes for Youth: Public Information-Gathering Session: Proceedings of a Workshop-In Brief*. Washington, DC: The National Academies Press.

O'Donnell, M.P. (2009). Definition of health promotion 2.0: Embracing passion, enhancing motivation, recognizing dynamic balance, and creating opportunities. *American Journal of Health Promotion, 24*(1), iv.

Onrust, S.A., Otten, R., Lammers, J., and Smit, F. (2016). School-based programmes to reduce and prevent substance use in different age groups: What works for whom? Systematic review and meta-regression analysis. *Clinical Psychology Review, 44*, 45–59.

Oringanje, C., Meremikwu, M.M., Eko, H., Esu, E., Meremikwu, A., and Ehiri, J.E. (2016). Interventions for preventing unintended pregnancies among adolescents. *Cochrane Database of Systematic Reviews*(2).

Pallmann, P., Bedding, A.W., Choodari-Oskooei, B., Dimairo, M., Flight, L., Hampson, L.V., Holmes, J., Mander, A.P., Odondi, L., Sydes, M.R., Villar, S.S., Wason, J.M.S., Weir, C.J., Wheeler, G.M., Yap, C., and Jaki, T. (2018). Adaptive designs in clinical trials: Why use them, and how to run and report them. *BMC Medicine, 16*(1), 29.

Peters, L.W.H., Kok, G., Ten Dam, G.T.M., Buijs, G.J., and Paulussen, T.G.W.M. (2009). Effective elements of school health promotion across behavioral domains: A systematic review of reviews. *BMC Public Health, 9*, 182.

Picot, J., Shepherd, J., Kavanagh, J., Cooper, K., Harden, A., Barnett-Page, E., Jones, J., Clegg, A., Hartwell, D., and Frampton, G.K. (2012). Behavioural interventions for the prevention of sexually transmitted infections in young people aged 13–19 years: A systematic review. *Health Education Research, 27*(3), 495–512.

Prochaska, J.O. and Velicer, W.F. (1997). The transtheoretical model of health behavior change. *American Journal of Health Promotion, 12*(1), 38–48.

San Diego Youth Services. (2019). *TPP Grantee Memo: San Diego Youth Services*. Memo to the Committee on Applying Lessons of Optimal Adolescent Health to Improve Behavioral Outcomes for Youth. San Diego, CA: San Diego Youth Services.

Seligman, L.D. and Ollendick, T.H. (2011). Cognitive-behavioral therapy for anxiety disorders in youth. *Child and Adolescent Psychiatric Clinics of North America, 20*(2), 217–238.

Seligman, M.E.P., and Csikszentmihalyi, M. (2014). Positive psychology: An introduction. In M. Csikszentmihalyi (Ed.), *Flow and the Foundations of Positive Psychology* (279–298). Berlin, Germany: Springer Science+Business Media.

Shepherd, J., Kavanagh, J., Picot, J., Cooper, K., Harden, A., Barnett-Page, E., Jones, J., Clegg, A., Hartwell, D., Frampton, G.K., and Price, A. (2010). The effectiveness and cost-effectiveness of behavioural interventions for the prevention of sexually transmitted infections in young people aged 13–19: A systematic review and economic evaluation. *Health Technology Assessment, 14*(7), 1–206, iii–iv.

Tanner-Smith, E.E., Steinka-Fry, K.T., Hennessy, E.A., Lipsey, M.W., and Winters, K.C. (2015). Can brief alcohol interventions for youth also address concurrent illicit drug use? Results from a meta-analysis. *Journal of Youth and Adolescence, 44*(5), 1011–1023.

Taylor, R.D., Oberle, E., Durlak, J.A., and Weissberg, R.P. (2017). Promoting positive youth development through school-based social and emotional learning interventions: A meta-analysis of follow-up effects. *Child Development, 88*(4), 1156–1171.

The Center for Black Women's Wellness Inc. (2019). *TPP Grantee Memo: The Center for Black Women's Wellness, Inc.* Memo to the Committee on Applying Lessons of Optimal Adolescent Health to Improve Behavioral Outcomes for Youth. Fulton County, GA: The Center for Black Women's Wellness, Inc.

Thomas, R.E., Lorenzetti, D.L., and Spragins, W. (2013). Systematic review of mentoring to prevent or reduce alcohol and drug use by adolescents. *Academic Pediatrics, 13*(4), 292–299.

Thomas, R.E., McLellan, J., and Perera, R. (2015). Effectiveness of school-based smoking prevention curricula: Systematic review and meta-analysis. *BMJ Open, 5*(3), e006976.

Tolan, P., Ross, K., Arkin, N., Godine, N., and Clark, E. (2016). Toward an integrated approach to positive development: Implications for intervention. *Applied Developmental Science, 20*(3), 214–236.

U.S. Department of Justice. (2013). *CrimeSolutions.gov Practices Scoring Instrument.* Washington, DC: Office of Justice Programs.

U.S. Preventive Services Task Force. (2018). *Procedure Manual.* Available: https://www.uspreventiveservicestaskforce.org/Page/Name/procedure-manual.

van Genugten, L., Dusseldorp, E., Massey, E.K., and van Empelen, P. (2017). Effective self-regulation change techniques to promote mental wellbeing among adolescents: A meta-analysis. *Health Psychology Review, 11*(1), 53–71.

Veritas Health Innovation. (2019). Covidence Systematic Review Software. Available: http://www.covidence.org.

Waters, E. and Sroufe, L.A. (1983). Social competence as a developmental construct. *Developmental Review, 3*(1), 79–97.

Whitaker, R., Hendry, M., Aslam, R.W., Booth, A., Carter, B., Charles, J.M., Craine, N., Edwards, R.T., Noyes, J., Ntambwe, L.I., Pasterfield, D., Rycroft-Malone, J., and Williams, N. (2016). Intervention now to eliminate repeat unintended pregnancy in teenagers (INTERUPT): A systematic review of intervention effectiveness and cost-effectiveness, and qualitative and realist synthesis of implementation factors and user engagement. *Health Technology Assessment, 20*(16), 1–214.

Wilson, S.J., Tanner-Smith, E.E., Lipsey, M.W., Steinka-Fry, K., and Morrison, J. (2011). Dropout prevention and intervention programs: Effects on school completion and dropout among school aged children and youth. *Campbell Systematic Reviews, 8*, 61.

5

Recommendations and Promising Approaches

Living my best life would be able to achieve my dreams and accomplishing the goals I've set for myself. Doing my best to past the obstacles in my path and never giving up along with supporting friends and family members. I would also say, living my best life would include having enough money to not worry about the total expenses used up each month.

Female, age 17[1]

The previous chapters of this report respond to the committee's charge to review key questions related to the effective implementation of youth programs. In particular, Chapter 2 examines the literature on adolescent development through an optimal health lens to set the stage for the review of programs in Chapter 4. Chapter 3 looks at adolescent risk taking and its social environmental influences, and provides an overview of the current landscape of the three specific behaviors (alcohol use, tobacco use, and sexual behavior) targeted by the committee for our program review. Chapter 4 then responds to the central charge to this committee—to use the optimal health framework to analyze the core components of programs found to be effective in preventing unhealthy risk behaviors among adolescents.

---

[1]Response to MyVoice survey question: "Describe what it would look like to live your best life." See the discussion of the MyVoice methodology in Appendix B for more detail.

This final chapter of the report synthesizes our findings and conclusions into recommendations and promising approaches for research, programs, and policies. In line with the charge in our statement of task to recommend (1) a research agenda incorporating a focus on optimal health for youth, and (2) improvements to the Office of the Assistant Secretary for Health's (OASH's) youth-focused programs, the three evidence-based recommendations presented in this chapter focus on the following:

- research on the effectiveness of core components of programs,
- updates to and expansion of data collection for the Youth Risk Behavior Survey (YRBS), and
- OASH programs.

We conclude with the following two promising approaches that, based on a broader examination of the contemporary research literature, represent significant opportunities for program improvement:

- policies and practices focused on inclusiveness and equity, and
- involvement of diverse youth in all decisions for youth programs.

RECOMMENDATIONS FOR RESEARCH

The two recommendations that respond to our charge to provide a research agenda incorporating a focus on optimal health for youth address (1) research on the effectiveness of core components of programs, and (2) updates to and expansion of data collection for the YRBS.

Research on the Effectiveness of Core Components of Programs

RECOMMENDATION 5-1: The U.S. Department of Health and Human Services should fund additional research aimed at identifying, measuring, and evaluating the effectiveness of specific core components of programs and interventions focused on promoting positive health behaviors and outcomes among adolescents.

Our recommendation for further research on the core components of programs is supported by the systematic review and examination of the literature on core components in Chapter 4.

Identification of the core components of evidence-based programs (EBPs) is a relatively new yet promising approach in the field of implementation science. As described in Chapter 4, this approach emerged from concerns about implementation fidelity to manualized or "name brand" EBPs for children's mental health conditions when a large number of "generic" programs without the EBP label had shown effectiveness in the community. In an attempt to broaden understanding of the effectiveness, relevance, and availability of evidence-based treatments, clinicians and researchers began undertaking clinical trials that deconstructed EBPs in order to identify their "active ingredients" (Blase and Fixsen, 2013). One example comes from studies of cognitive-behavioral therapy (CBT), one of the most widely used and effective interventions for internalizing problems. Core components research on CBT has shown that exposure to a fear or stressor may be the most important component of this therapy for anxiety and traumatic stress (Seligman and Ollendick, 2011). Moreover, distilling treatments into their active components can help reduce the length of interventions, which in turn can increase treatment fidelity, compliance, and access for diverse populations.

More recent research on the core components of programs for adolescents has shown the utility of this approach with respect to not only mental health, but also opioid use disorder (OUD) and youth program management and quality improvement. For example, researchers at the Center on Addiction have been able to identify 21 core techniques focused on family psychoeducation, medication options, and shared decision making that are most effective for youth in OUD treatment (National Academies of Sciences, Engineering, and Medicine [NASEM], 2019a). With regard to program management and quality improvement, a team at the David P. Weikart Center for Youth Program Quality conducted a systematic review and meta-analysis to identify high-quality practices that could be used by youth workers to promote positive outcomes among youth in after-school programs. Applying the results of this research, they created the Youth Program Quality Assessment, which can be used to measure program quality and identify staff training needs (NASEM, 2019a).

Three main methods can be used to identify core components of programs (see Chapter 4). The first is the distillation and matching method (used by Boustani et al., 2015), which aims to identify the distinct techniques within a treatment that can be used to individualize services (Chorpita, Daleiden, and Weisz, 2005). The second method is the Delphi technique, which involves convening focus groups of experts to reach consensus on the most effective components of a set of treatments (Garland et al., 2008). The third method is meta-analysis and meta-regression (used by Hahn et al., 2015; Wilson et al., 2011; Tanner-Smith et al., 2015), which applies quantitative methods to analyze the relative effectiveness of program components (Lipsey, 2018).

While all of these methods can help identify common components of effective programs, not all are designed to test their *effectiveness*. To address the issue of effectiveness, several efforts have focused on implementing core components approaches in practice settings and evaluating whether the use of these methods is associated with better outcomes. Examples include Chorpita et al. (2013, 2017) for children's mental health; Smith et al. (2012) for after-school programs; and Lipsey (2008), Lipsey, Howell, and Tidd (2007), and Redpath and Brandner (2010) for juvenile delinquency. These examples show promise for core components approaches, but these approaches have not yet been validated for adolescent health behaviors and outcomes more broadly. Therefore, we recommend that the U.S. Department of Health and Human Services (HHS) fund research focused on further exploring the use of core components approaches to identify the components of effective programs that promote adolescent health and test whether those components do in fact result in better health outcomes. If so, these components could be used to develop shorter and more focused interventions that would be (1) less costly and require less facilitator training, which could lead to greater program fidelity, and (2) more accessible to diverse populations.

Updates to and Expansion of the Youth Risk Behavior Survey

RECOMMENDATION 5-2: The Division of Adolescent and School Health of the Centers for Disease Control and Prevention should

- **update and expand the Youth Risk Behavior Survey (YRBS) to include**
  - **out-of-school youth (e.g., homeless, incarcerated, dropped out), and**
  - **survey items that reflect a more comprehensive set of sexual risk behaviors with specific definitions; and**
- **conduct further research on the ideal setting and mode for administering the YRBS with today's adolescents.**

As described in Chapters 1 and 3, we chose to use the YRBS to describe trends in adolescent risk behavior because it (1) covers all three of our behaviors of interest, and (2) is the dataset used most often by the sponsor to evaluate youth risk behavior trends. However, our use of YRBS data in this report by no means suggests that these data are perfect. We therefore believe there are specific actions that the Centers for Disease Control and Prevention (CDC) can take to provide a more accurate picture of trends in adolescent risk behavior moving forward.

First and foremost, we recommend that the YRBS begin including out-of-school youth in the sampling design. Although the YRBS estimates that out-of-school adolescents represent only 3 percent of the adolescent population, other research suggests that this figure could be as high as 10.1 percent

(Brener et al., 2013; King, Marino, and Barry, 2018). This population is especially important because those adolescents who are not in school, particularly those who are homeless or incarcerated or have dropped out, have higher incidences of the risk behaviors addressed in this report and their related adverse health outcomes compared with those who are in school (Edidin et al., 2012; Freudenberg and Ruglis, 2007; Heitzeg, 2009; Kearney and Levine, 2012; Odgers, Robins, and Russell, 2010; Tolou-Shams et al., 2019; Wilson et al., 2011). An updated and expanded YRBS that captured data on these youth could help inform programs and interventions for these marginalized groups of adolescents.

Second, we recommend updating the sexual behavior items on the YRBS to reflect the variety of sexual behaviors in which today's youth engage. The survey's current sexual behavior questions are vague, referring to "sexual intercourse" without providing a clear definition of this term. Most of the subsequent questions also tend to focus on pregnancy risk, which further suggests that "sexual intercourse" refers only to penile–vaginal intercourse. This wording is inherently flawed for multiple reasons. First, today's adolescents have different conceptualizations of sex and sexual activity relative to their counterparts in the past (Diamond and Savin-Williams, 2009). Accordingly, respondents may interpret "sexual intercourse" to mean any type of sex (vaginal, oral, or anal) and/or to include only consensual sexual activity, which can lead to biased estimates of the behavior of interest. Second, the emphasis on vaginal sex and pregnancy risk ignores the impact of sexually transmitted infections (STIs), whose incidence is disproportionately higher in adolescents and young adults compared with adult populations (CDC, 2018). Similarly, the focus on vaginal sex excludes LGBTQ adolescents, who are primarily at risk for STIs and may never engage in penile-vaginal intercourse. We therefore recommend that future YRBS cycles not only include a definition for "sexual intercourse," but also ask about experiences of vaginal, oral, and anal sex in order to provide a more accurate picture of adolescent sexual risk.

Fortunately, the CDC does not have to start from scratch. Other nationally representative surveys, including the National Survey of Family Growth (NSFG), have successfully implemented these types of questions with adolescent populations. Appendix C shows the comparable items on the YRBS and NSFG, which can be used to identify appropriate oral and anal sex questions as well as example definitions for each of these behaviors.

Thus, by implementing the aforementioned changes to the sampling design and sexual behavior items, the YRBS will be able to provide estimates that are more (1) representative of the entire U.S. adolescent population, (2) precise, and (3) reflective of contemporary behavior trends. As a result, these data can be used to make sure that adolescent health programs and interventions are reflective of the behavior trends and needs of today's youth.

Finally, we recommend that the CDC conduct further research regarding the ideal setting and mode for administering the YRBS with contemporary cohorts of youth. As described in Chapter 3, the most recent evaluation of YRBS setting and mode effects was conducted in 2008 (Brener et al., 2013; Denniston et al., 2010; Eaton et al., 2010). However, the technological landscape over the last decade has changed significantly, particularly among adolescents. For example, as described in Chapter 2, 95 percent of today's youth have a smartphone, ranging from 93 percent among those with a household income of $30,000 or less to 97 percent among those with a household income of $75,000 or more (Anderson and Jiang, 2018). As a result, a web-based survey mode may be more effective than paper-and-pencil instruments for today's youth. Furthermore, if shown to be effective, a web-based survey could also make the YRBS more accessible to out-of-school youth, as described above.

RECOMMENDATION FOR OASH PROGRAMS

This section of the chapter presents our recommendation for OASH programs. Specifically, this recommendation responds to the statement of task for this study by providing ways that OASH can use its role to foster the adoption of promising elements of youth focused programs in the initiatives it oversees, such as those focused on mental and physical health, adolescent development, and reproductive health and teen pregnancy.

RECOMMENDATION 5-3: The Office of the Assistant Secretary for Health within the U.S. Department of Health and Human Services should fund universal, holistic, multicomponent programs that meet all of the following criteria:

- **promote and improve the health and well-being of the whole person, laying the foundation for specific, developmentally appropriate behavioral skills development;**
- **begin in early childhood and are offered during critical developmental windows, from childhood throughout adolescence;**
- **consider adolescent decision making, exploration, and risk taking as normative;**
- **engage diverse communities, public policy makers, and societal leaders to improve modifiable social and environmental determinants of health and well-being that disadvantage and stress young people and their families; and**
- **are theory driven and evidence based.**

This recommendation is grounded in the findings from our systematic review and examination of core components papers presented in Chapter 4. Although we reviewed programs targeting individual behaviors (e.g., substance use, sexual behavior), application of the optimal health framework revealed an important and heretofore neglected area of investment: broadening the focus of OASH-funded programs to teach skills that, if learned successfully, underlie and impact health and well-being across the life course (see Klingbeil et al., 2017). Specifically, evidence shows that integrating and coordinating funding for programs that focus on social-emotional learning and positive youth development would be more effective in targeting adolescent health behaviors and related outcomes relative to the fragmented approach taken in the past (Taylor et al., 2017; U.S. Department of Health and Human Services, 2018). Our review also showed the strengths of social-emotional learning programs initiated in early childhood and continued through adolescence (Taylor et al., 2017), particularly in demonstrating that the nature of the positive effects of such programs may differ across developmental stages (Dray et al., 2017).

It must be emphasized that this recommendation for universal social-emotional learning and positive youth development programs should not be taken as a suggestion that programs targeting specific health behaviors (e.g., substance abuse prevention, inclusive sex education) are not important. Rather, we view the more holistic programs recommended here as building a foundation of self-regulation, good decision making, social awareness, and relationship skills upon which other specific behavioral skills and services (e.g., understanding social norms around drugs, negotiating condom use, access to contraception) can be built.

This recommendation is also informed by our review of the literature on adolescent risk taking in Chapter 3, where we draw a critical distinction between healthy and unhealthy risk taking. Healthy risk taking is a normal and necessary part of adolescent identity development, providing adolescents with opportunities to explore their environments, practice decision-making skills, and develop autonomy. In contrast, unhealthy risk-taking behaviors are often illegal or dangerous, and may result in adverse health outcomes that impede adolescent development. Therefore, instead of conceptualizing all risk taking as negative, it is important to acknowledge its developmental purpose and provide opportunities for adolescents to take healthy risks that will help them learn, grow, and thrive.

Our recommendation for OASH programs also reflects the critical importance of reducing health disparities and promoting health equity by targeting the social determinants of health that disadvantage marginalized communities. As mentioned throughout this and other National Academies reports, marginalized adolescents (e.g., homeless, justice-involved, estranged from their families, identifying as LGBTQ, having a disability), particularly those who are racially and ethnically diverse and/or from lower-income groups, need more resources relative to their peers from more advantaged backgrounds (Auerswald, Piatt, and Mirzazadeh, 2017; NASEM, 2017, 2019b). Moreover, when standardized programs are implemented in these communities, they often fail to meet the needs of the youth who are targeted. It is therefore critical that OASH programs continue to be developed and implemented with input and support from the communities they serve, as those insights will help identify the most pressing needs for the respective youth populations.

Finally, we recommend that these programs be theory-based and informed by scientific research evidence. Regarding the current research base, our review of programs in Chapter 4 indicates that effective approaches are more likely to be theory-based, to address social influences and norms, to incorporate cognitive-behavioral skills, and to consist of multiple components. However, recognizing that much of the research documented in the current scientific literature was not designed to evaluate the effectiveness of core program components, we recommend that these programs continue to evolve based on future research (see Recommendation 5-1). By continuing to rely on the most up-to-date scientific evidence, OASH will be better positioned to continuously improve the youth programs and initiatives it oversees.

PROMISING APPROACHES

As stated earlier, the committee's ability to identify core components of programs was hindered by the limited number of studies in the literature that were designed to examine the effectiveness of specific components. However, in line with the charge in our statement of task to identify promising elements of youth-focused programs, we are suggesting two approaches that deserve meaningful attention in the design, implementation, and evaluation of adolescent health programs.

Promoting Inclusiveness and Equity

PROMISING APPROACH 5-1: Programs can benefit from implementing and evaluating policies and practices that promote inclusiveness and equity so that all youth are able to thrive.

Our first promising approach relates to OASH's role in convening, coordinating, and driving policy and policy discussions. As mentioned in Recommendation 5-3, targeting the social determinants of health that disadvantage marginalized communities is critically important for reducing health disparities and promoting health equity in adolescent health programs. However, beyond focusing programmatic efforts toward communities with the greatest need, *all* health education programs can benefit from implementing policies and practices that promote cultural inclusiveness and equity. In particular, programs need to address the structural inequities, including racism, sexism, classism, ableism, xenophobia, and homophobia, that lead to health inequities. When programs are not inclusive and equitable, they can be discriminatory, leading to worse overall outcomes that are both unfair and avoidable (NASEM, 2017; Williams and Mohammed, 2013). Thus, implementing these policies and practices in all programs can avoid the systematic and counterproductive exclusion of youth who may benefit from those programs.

As described by the CDC, an effective health education curriculum "incorporates learning strategies, teaching methods, and materials that are culturally inclusive" (2019). Such practices include (CDC, 2019, para. 13)

- using materials that are free of culturally biased information;
- incorporating information, activities, and examples that are inclusive of diverse cultures and lifestyles (such as genders, races, ethnicities, religions, ages, physical/mental abilities, appearances, and sexual orientations);
- promoting values, attitudes, and behaviors that acknowledge the cultural diversity of students;
- optimizing relevance to students from multiple cultures in the school community;
- strengthening the skills students need to engage in intercultural interactions; and
- building on the cultural resources of families and communities.

Importantly, beyond encouraging programs to adopt specific policies and practices that promote equity and inclusion, these aspects of programs need to be formally evaluated. Although our review of programs as documented in Chapter 4 yielded some evidence that a supportive and inclusive culture improves program effectiveness, the extent to which programs included in our review had such policies or used such practices was rarely if ever measured. We recognize, however, that the limited evidence from our review is due more likely to the constraints of our statement of task and our systematic review methodology than to the relevance of these policies and practices for youth programs.

A variety of resources and tools are available that can help organizations plan, implement, and evaluate culturally and linguistically competent policies and practices. For example, the National Center for Cultural Competence at Georgetown University provides an extensive literature and a number of training and self-assessment tools that can be used to inform, monitor, and improve the cultural and linguistic competency of organizations and programs, particularly those that work with children and adolescents.[2] By using these and other resources, OASH can promote program effectiveness by ensuring the implementation and evaluation of policies and practices focused on equity and inclusion in all of the initiatives it oversees.

Youth Involvement

PROMISING APPROACH 5-2: Programs can benefit from including youth of diverse ages, racial/ethnic backgrounds, socioeconomic status, rurality/urbanity, sexual orientations, sexes/genders, and disability/ability status in their decision-making processes.

Partnering with diverse youth in the development of policies and programs that impact their health and well-being is critical to ensure the success of these programs (OECD, 2017). Youth are experts in their own experiences and challenges (Wyatt and Oliver, 2016), and as discussed in Chapters 2 and 3, this particular generation has experienced a number of rapid technological and cultural changes that have affected not only how they interact but also how they access and process information about their health. Understanding these experiences is pivotal in creating policies that address and alleviate barriers to promoting their health.

If they become engaged in policy making, youth can openly express their preferences and needs. Evidence from community-based participatory research demonstrates that engaging target populations as full and equal partners ensures that their needs, preferences, and values are reflected in policies and programs designed to impact their well-being (Holkup et al., 2004; Murry and Brody, 2004; Wallerstein et al., 2015). Moreover, including youth from diverse age groups (early, middle, late adolescence), racial/ethnic backgrounds, socioeconomic status, rurality/urbanity, sexual orientations, sexes/genders, and disability/ability status from the very beginning of program development can help make these programs more acceptable and effective for the diverse groups they serve (Ford, Rasmus, and Allen, 2012; Mirra and Garcia, 2017; OECD, 2017; Powers and Tiffany, 2006).

Civic engagement of youth enhances the effectiveness of public policy; conversely, the success of programs and policies is undermined when researchers and policy makers do not authentically value the expertise of youth (OECD, 2017). Promoting participation by youth increases their ownership of policies and programs, which is essential for success, while

---

[2]For more information on the National Center for Cultural Competence, see https://nccc.georgetown.edu.

also building consensus on key policies. This participation can lead to more effective policy implementation and also strengthen the relationship between citizens and government (Partridge et al., 2018). Thus, engaging youth as experts can yield reciprocal benefits for youth, researchers, and policy makers (Zeldin, Christens, and Powers, 2013).

Given its role as a leader in adolescent health policy at the national level, OASH has a unique opportunity to engage with youth on the issues that affect them. By involving youth in its decision-making processes, OASH can capitalize on their knowledge and experiences to improve its youth-focused programs while also providing positive youth development opportunities for the young people involved in this process.

REFERENCES

Anderson, M. and Jiang, J. (2018). *Teens, Social Media & Technology 2018*. Washington, DC: Pew Research Center.

Auerswald, C.L., Piatt, A.A., and Mirzazadeh, A. (2017). *Research with Disadvantaged, Vulnerable and/or Marginalized Adolescents*. Florence, Italy: UNICEF Office of Research.

Blase, K., and Fixsen, D. (2013). Core intervention components: Identifying and operationalizing what makes programs work. *ASPE Research Brief*. U.S. Department of Health and Human Services. Available: https://aspe.hhs.gov/report/core-intervention-components-identifying-and-operationalizing-what-makes-programs-work.

Boustani, M.M., Frazier, S.L., Becker, K.D., Bechor, M., Dinizulu, S.M., Hedemann, E.R., Ogle, R.R., and Pasalich, D.S. (2015). Common elements of adolescent prevention programs: Minimizing burden while maximizing reach. *Administration and Policy in Mental Health and Mental Health Services Research*, 42(2), 209–219.

Brener, N.D., Kann, L., Shanklin, S., Kinchen, S., Eaton, D.K., Hawkins, J., and Flint, K.H. (2013). Methodology of the Youth Risk Behavior Surveillance System—2013. *Morbidity and Mortality Weekly Report: Recommendations and Reports*, 62(1), 1–20.

Centers for Disease Control and Prevention. (2018). STDs in adolescents and young adults. *Sexually Transmitted Disease Surveillance 2017: Special Focus Profiles*. Available: https://www.cdc.gov/std/stats17/adolescents.htm.

Centers for Disease Control and Prevention (2019). *Characteristics of an Effective Health Education Curriculum*. Available: https://www.cdc.gov/healthyschools/sher/characteristics/index.htm.

Chorpita, B.F., Daleiden, E.L., and Weisz, J.R. (2005). Identifying and selecting the common elements of evidence based interventions: A distillation and matching model. *Mental Health Services Research*, 7(1), 5–20.

Chorpita, B.F., Weisz, J.R., Daleiden, E.L., Schoenwald, S.K., Palinkas, L.A., Miranda, J., Higa-McMillan, C.K., Nakamura, B.J., Austin, A.A., and Borntrager, C.F. (2013). Long-term outcomes for the Child STEPs randomized effectiveness trial: A comparison of modular and standard treatment designs with usual care. *Journal of Consulting and Clinical Psychology*, 81(6), 999.

Chorpita, B.F., Daleiden, E.L., Park, A.L., Ward, A.M., Levy, M.C., Cromley, T., Chiu, A.W., Letamendi, A.M., Tsai, K.H., and Krull, J.L. (2017). Child STEPs in California: A cluster randomized effectiveness trial comparing modular treatment with community implemented treatment for youth with anxiety, depression, conduct problems, or traumatic stress. *Journal of Consulting and Clinical Psychology*, 85(1), 13.

Denniston, M.M., Brener, N.D., Kann, L., Eaton, D.K., McManus, T., Kyle, T.M., Roberts, A.M., Flint, K.H., and Ross, J.G. (2010). Comparison of paper-and-pencil versus web administration of the Youth Risk Behavior Survey (YRBS): Participation, data quality, and perceived privacy and anonymity. *Computers in Human Behavior, 26*(5), 1054–1060.

Diamond, L.M., and Savin-Williams, R.C. (2009). Adolescent sexuality. In R.M. Lerner and L. Steinberg (Eds.), *Handbook of Adolescent Psychology: Individual Bases of Adolescent Development* (pp. 479–524). Hoboken, NJ: John Wiley & Sons, Inc.

Dray, J., Bowman, J., Campbell, E., Freund, M., Wolfenden, L., Hodder, R.K., McElwaine, K., Tremain, D., Bartlem, K., Bailey, J., Small, T., Palazzi, K., Oldmeadow, C., and Wiggers, J. (2017). Systematic review of universal resilience-focused interventions targeting child and adolescent mental health in the school setting. *Journal of the American Academy of Child & Adolescent Psychiatry, 56*(10), 813–824.

Eaton, D.K., Brener, N.D., Kann, L., Denniston, M.M., McManus, T., Kyle, T.M., Roberts, A.M., Flint, K.H., and Ross, J.G. (2010). Comparison of paper-and-pencil versus web administration of the Youth Risk Behavior Survey (YRBS): Risk behavior prevalence estimates. *Evaluation Review, 34*(2), 137–153.

Edidin, J.P., Ganim, Z., Hunter, S.J., and Karnik, N.S. (2012). The mental and physical health of homeless youth: A literature review. *Child Psychiatry & Human Development, 43*(3), 354-375.

Ford, T., Rasmus, S., and Allen, J. (2012). Being useful: Achieving indigenous youth involvement in a community-based participatory research project in Alaska. *International Journal of Circumpolar Health, 71*(1), 18413.

Freudenberg, N., and Ruglis, J. (2007). Reframing school dropout as a public health issue. *Preventing Chronic Disease: Public Health Research, Practice, and Policy, 4*(4).

Garland, A.F., Hawley, K.M., Brookman-Frazee, L., and Hurlburt, M.S. (2008). Identifying common elements of evidence-based psychosocial treatments for children's disruptive behavior problems. *Journal of the American Academy of Child & Adolescent Psychiatry, 47*(5), 505–514.

Hahn, R.A., Knopf, J.A., Wilson, S.J., Truman, B.I., Milstein, B., Johnson, R.L., Fielding, J.E., Muntaner, C.J.M., Jones, C.P., Fullilove, M.T., Moss, R.D., Ueffing, E., and Hunt, P.C. (2015). Programs to increase high school completion: A Community Guide systematic health equity review. *American Journal of Preventive Medicine, 48*(5), 599–608.

Heitzeg, N.A. (2009). Education or incarceration: Zero tolerance policies and the school to prison pipeline. *Forum on Public Policy, 9*(2).

Holkup, P.A., Tripp-Reimer, T., Salois, E.M., and Weinert, C. (2004). Community-based participatory research: An approach to intervention research with a Native American community. *Advances in Nursing Science, 27*(3), 162.

Kearney, M.S., and Levine, P.B. (2012). Why is the teen birth rate in the United States so high and why does it matter? *Journal of Economic Perspectives, 26*(2), 141–163.

King, B.M., Marino, L.E., and Barry, K.R. (2018). Does the Centers for Disease Control and Prevention's Youth Risk Behavior Survey underreport risky sexual behavior? *Sexually Transmitted Diseases, 45*(3), e10–e11.

Klingbeil, D.A., Renshaw, T.L., Willenbrink, J.B., Copek, R.A., Chan, K.T., Haddock, A., Yassine, J., and Clifton, J. (2017). Mindfulness-based interventions with youth: A comprehensive meta-analysis of group-design studies. *Journal of School Psychology, 63*, 77–103.

Lipsey, M.W. (2008). *The Arizona Standardized Program Evaluation Protocol (SPEP) for Assessing the Effectiveness of Programs for Juvenile Probationers: SPEP Ratings and Relative Recidivism Reduction for the Initial SPEP Sample.* Nashville, TN: Vanderbilt University Center for Evaluation Research and Methodology.

Lipsey, M.W. (2018). Effective use of the large body of research on the effectiveness of programs for juvenile offenders and the failure of the model programs approach. *Criminology & Public Policy, 17*(1), 189–198.

Lipsey, M.W., Howell, J.C., and Tidd, S.T. (2007). *The Standardized Program Evaluation Protocol (SPEP): A Practical Approach to Evaluating and Improving Juvenile Justice Programs in North Carolina. Final Evaluation Report.* Nashville, TN: Vanderbilt University Center for Evaluation Research and Methodology.

Mirra, N., and Garcia, A. (2017). Civic participation reimagined: Youth interrogation and innovation in the multimodal public sphere. *Review of Research in Education, 41*(1), 136–158.

Murry, V.M. and Brody, G.H. (2004). Partnering with community stakeholders: Engaging rural African American families in basic research and The Strong African American Families Preventive Intervention Program. *Journal of Marital and Family Therapy, 30*(3), 271–283.

National Academies of Sciences, Engineering, and Medicine (NASEM). (2017). *Communities in Action: Pathways to Health Equity.* Washington, DC: The National Academies Press.

———. (2019a). *Applying Lessons of Optimal Adolescent Health to Improve Behavioral Outcomes for Youth: Public Information-Gathering Session: Proceedings of a Workshop-in-Brief.* Washington, DC: The National Academies Press.

———. (2019b). *The Promise of Adolescence: Realizing Opportunity for All Youth.* Washington, DC: The National Academies Press.

Odgers, C.L., Robins, S.J., and Russell, M.A. (2010). Morbidity and mortality risk among the "forgotten few": Why are girls in the justice system in such poor health? *Law and Human Behavior, 34*(6), 429–444.

Organisation for Economic Co-operation and Development. (2017). Engaging youth in policy-making processes (Module 6). *Evidence-Based Policy Making for Youth Well-Being: A Toolkit.* Paris, France: OECD Publishing.

Partridge, L., Astle, J., Grinsted, S., and Strong, F.L. (2018). *Teenagency: How Young People Can Create a Better World.* London, England: Royal Society for the Encouragement of Arts, Manufactures and Commerce.

Powers, J.L. and Tiffany, J.S. (2006). Engaging youth in participatory research and evaluation. *Journal of Public Health Management and Practice, 12,* S79–S87.

Redpath, D.P. and Brandner, J.K. (2010). *The Arizona Standardized Program Evaluation Protocol (SPEP) for Assessing the Effectiveness of Programs for Juvenile Probationers: SPEP Rating and Relative Recidivism Reduction; An Update to the January 2008 Report by Dr. Mark Lipsey.* Phoenix, AZ: Arizona Supreme Court, Administrative Office of the Courts, Juvenile Justice Service Division.

Seligman, L.D. and Ollendick, T.H. (2011). Cognitive-behavioral therapy for anxiety disorders in youth. *Child and Adolescent Psychiatric Clinics of North America, 20*(2), 217–238.

Smith, C., Akiva, T., Sugar, S., Lo, Y.-J., Frank, K., Peck, S.C., Cortina, K.S., and Devaney, T. (2012). *Continuous Quality Improvement in Afterschool Settings: Impact Findings from the Youth Program Quality Intervention Study.* Washington, DC: The Forum for Youth Investment.

Tanner-Smith, E.E., Steinka-Fry, K.T., Hennessy, E.A., Lipsey, M.W., and Winters, K.C. (2015). Can brief alcohol interventions for youth also address concurrent illicit drug use? Results from a meta-analysis. *Journal of Youth and Adolescence, 44*(5), 1011–1023.

Taylor, R.D., Oberle, E., Durlak, J.A., and Weissberg, R.P. (2017). Promoting positive youth development through school-based social and emotional learning interventions: A meta-analysis of follow-up effects. *Child Development, 88*(4), 1156–1171.

Tolou-Shams, M., Harrison, A., Hirschtritt, M.E., Dauria, E., and Barr-Walker, J. (2019). Substance use and HIV among justice-involved youth: Intersecting risks. *Current HIV/AIDS Reports, 16*(1), 37-47.

U.S. Department of Health and Human Services. (2018). *Adolescent Health: Think, Act, Grow® Playbook.* Washington, DC: U.S. Department of Health and Human Services, Office of Population Affairs, Office of Adolescent Health.

Wallerstein, N., Minkler, M., Carter-Edwards, L., Avila, M., and Sanchez, V. (2015). Improving health through community engagement, community organization, and community building. In K. Glanz, B.K. Rimer and K. Viswanath (Eds.), *Health Behavior: Theory, Research and Practice* (5th ed., pp. 277–300). San Francisco, CA: Jossey-Bass.

Williams, D.R. and Mohammed, S.A. (2013). Racism and health I: Pathways and scientific evidence. *American Behavioral Scientist, 57*(8), 1152–1173.

Wilson, S.J., Tanner-Smith, E.E., Lipsey, M.W., Steinka-Fry, K., and Morrison, J. (2011). Dropout prevention and intervention programs: Effects on school completion and dropout among school aged children and youth. *Campbell Systematic Reviews, 8*, 61.

Wyatt, Z. and Oliver, L. (2016). Y-change: Young people as experts and collaborators. *Advances in Social Work and Welfare Education, 18*(1), 121.

Zeldin, S., Christens, B.D., and Powers, J.L. (2013). The psychology and practice of youth-adult partnership: Bridging generations for youth development and community change. *American Journal of Community Psychology, 51*(3–4), 385–397.

Appendix A

Literature Search Strategy

A professional research librarian from the National Academies of Sciences, Engineering, and Medicine conducted a comprehensive literature search for this study based on the statement of task and reference interviews with program staff to identify relevant research on optimal adolescent health. Electronic literature searches of systematic reviews and meta-analyses published between 2009 and 2019 were conducted in the following electronic bibliographic databases: Cochrane Database of Systematic Reviews, Campbell Collaboration Library, PubMed, and PsycINFO. The inclusion/exclusion criteria for the search are shown in Table A-1.

The search terms were adapted to each database, and separate searches were conducted around the different domains of optimal adolescent health. Generally, three blocks of terms were used: one describing the sample or population of interest (e.g., teens, adolescents), one describing the optimal adolescent health domain or subdomain of interest (e.g., sexual risk behavior, pregnancy), and one identifying meta-analyses and systematic reviews. Table A-2 lists the literature search topics; Table A-3 provides the search terms used; and Table A-4 gives an example of search term combinations from the search of the Cochrane Database of Systematic Reviews.

TABLE A-1 Inclusion/Exclusion Criteria

Inclusion Criteria	Exclusion Criteria
Publication year: 2009–present	Publication year: Before 2009
Available in English: Yes	Unavailable in English
Peer-reviewed articles: Yes	Publications other than peer-reviewed articles
Age range: 10–19	Age range: other than 10–19

TABLE A-2 Search Topics

Topic	Date	Literature	Date Range	Databases
Physical Health • Substance Use • Sexual Behavior	04/15/2019	Systematic Reviews, Meta-analysis	2009-Present	Cochrane Database of Systematic Reviews, Campbell Collaboration Library, PubMed, and PsycINFO
Emotional Health	05/07/2019	Systematic Reviews, Meta-analysis	2009-Present	Cochrane Database of Systematic Reviews, Campbell Collaboration Library, PubMed, and PsycINFO
Social Health	05/07/2019	Systematic Reviews, Meta-analysis	2009-Present	Cochrane Database of Systematic Reviews, Campbell Collaboration Library, PubMed, and PsycINFO
Spiritual Health	05/07/2019	Systematic Reviews, Meta-analysis	2009-Present	Cochrane Database of Systematic Reviews, Campbell Collaboration Library, PubMed, and PsycINFO
Intellectual Health	05/07/2019	Systematic Reviews, Meta-analysis	2009-Present	Cochrane Database of Systematic Reviews, Campbell Collaboration Library, PubMed, and PsycINFO

TABLE A-3 Search Terms

Preliminary Terms	Indexing Terms

1. Teenagers
  1.1 adolescent
  1.2 age range: 10 to 19
  1.3 teen
  1.4 teenager
	adolescent (MeSH)
	
	KEYWORDS
	adolescent
	teen
	teenager
	youth

2. Teenage Pregnancy
  2.1 abstinence
  2.2 comprehensive sexual education
  2.3 youth development
  2.4 teenage pregnancy prevention
	sexual abstinence (MeSH)
	sex education (MeSH)
	pregnancy in adolescence/prevention &
	  control (MeSH)
	
	KEYWORDS
	celibacy
	comprehensive sexual education
	youth development
	adolescent pregnancy prevention
	teen pregnancy prevention
	teenage pregnancy prevention

3. Reproductive Health
  3.1 contraception
  3.2 STI screening and treatment
  3.3 healthy pregnancy care and services
  3.4 hpv vaccination
  3.5 general preventive healthcare
	contraception (MeSH)
	sexually transmitted diseases/prevention &
	  control (MeSH)
	sexually transmitted diseases/therapy
	  (MeSH)
	pregnancy in adolescence (MeSH)
	adolescent health services (MeSH)
	health services (MeSH)
	papillomavirus vaccines (MeSH)
	preventive health services (MeSH)
	preventive medicine (MeSH)
	
	KEYWORDS
	hpv vaccines
	human papilloma virus vaccines

continued

TABLE A-3 Continued

Preliminary Terms	Indexing Terms

4. Substance Use Prevention
   4.1 alcohol
   4.2 tobacco
      4.2.1 e-cigarettes
   4.3 illicit drugs
      4.3.1 cannabis
	alcohol drinking/prevention & control (MeSH)
	binge drinking/prevention & control (MeSH)
	underage drinking/prevention & control (MeSH)
	alcohol abstinence (MeSH)
	temperance (MeSH)
	cigarette smoking/prevention & control (MeSH)
	smoking/prevention & control (MeSH)
	vaping/prevention & control (MeSH)
	anti-smoking campaign (MeSH)
	anti-smoking education (MeSH)
	smoking cessation (MeSH)
	smoking prevention (MeSH)
	tobacco use cessation (MeSH)
	marijuana smoking/prevention & control (MeSH)
	street drugs/prevention & control (MeSH)
	substance-related disorders/prevention & control (MeSH)
	risk reduction behavior (MeSH)

	KEYWORDS teenage drinking smoking vaping cannabis smoking drug abuse drug addiction illicit drugs recreational drugs substance abuse

5. Emotional Health
   5.1 resilience
   5.2 mental health
   5.3 emotion regulation
   5.4 self-regulation
   5.5 stress management
	mental health (MeSH)
	relaxation therapy (MeSH)

	KEYWORDS emotional well-being psychological well-being social well-being mental hygiene mental health emotional resilience emotional self-regulation emotion regulation stress management

TABLE A-3 Continued

Preliminary Terms	Indexing Terms
6. Social Health 6.1 social emotional learning 6.2 conflict resolution 6.3 assertiveness 6.4 social skills	social learning (MeSH) assertiveness (MeSH) negotiating (MeSH) social skills (MeSH)
	KEYWORDS social health social and emotional learning conflict resolution mediation interpersonal skills social abilities social competence
7. Intellectual Health 7.1 academic achievement 7.2 afterschool 7.3 academic performance 7.4 learning 7.5 mentoring	academic success (MeSH) academic performance (MeSH) achievement (MeSH) learning (MeSH) mentoring (MeSH)
	KEYWORDS intellectual health academic achievement afterschool academic test scores educational test performance educational test scores coaching
8. Spiritual Health 8.1 mindfulness 8.2 character education 8.3 values education	mindfulness (MeSH) moral development (MeSH)
	KEYWORDS spiritual health character education values education
9. Intervention 9.1 program(s) (programme(s)) 9.2 intervention(s) 9.3 treatment(s) 9.4 therapy (therapies)	government programs (MeSH) therapeutics (MeSH)
	KEYWORDS intervention program programmes treatment therapy
10. Type 10.1 meta-analysis 10.2 systematic review	meta-analysis (MeSH) systematic review (MeSH)

TABLE A-4 Example of Search Combinations

1	(adolescent$1 or teen$1 or teenager$1 or youth or underage or young).ti. or (adolescent$1 or teen$1 or teenager$1 or youth or underage or young).ab. or (adolescent$1 or teen$1 or teenager$1 or youth or underage or young).kw.
2	(smoking or vaping or tobacco).ti. or (smoking or vaping or tobacco).ab. or (smoking or vaping or tobacco).kw.
3	("cannabis smoking" or "drug abuse" or "drug addiction" or "illicit drugs" or "recreational drugs" or "substance abuse").ti. or ("cannabis smoking" or "drug abuse" or "drug addiction" or "illicit drugs" or "recreational drugs" or "substance abuse").ab. or ("cannabis smoking" or "drug abuse" or "drug addiction" or "illicit drugs" or "recreational drugs" or "substance abuse").kw.
4	(prevent$3 or anti?smoking or cessation).mp.
5	2 and 3
6	4 and 5
7	1 and 6
8	limit 7 to last 10 years

Appendix B

MyVoice Methodology

The MyVoice study is an interactive research platform from the University of Michigan that sends out weekly surveys to adolescents ages 14–24 via text message. Each survey focuses on a different topic and includes three to five brief, open-ended questions.

In August 2019, the committee commissioned MyVoice to conduct a poll of its sample on what it means for youth to thrive. The original questions were workshopped and piloted with a group of adolescents on the MyVoice leadership team, who suggested using the phrase "live your best life" as a synonym for thrive.

The resulting four questions were sent to the MyVoice sample, from which 945 unique responses were received:

- *Hi {{name}}! This week we want to hear about what it means to be a thriving young person. Describe what it would look like to live your best life.*
- *Tell us about something or someone that helps you live your best life.*
- *Specifically, what could your school do to help you live your best life (now or in the past)?*
- *What keeps you from living your best life, if anything?*

The full commissioned paper from MyVoice is available in the online appendixes to this consensus report.[1]

---

[1]For more information, see MyVoice (2019) (https://www.hearmyvoicenow.org).

Appendix C

Comparison of
Youth Risk Behavior Survey (YRBS) and
National Survey of Family Growth (NSFG)
Survey Items on Sexual Behavior

Question Category	YRBS Questionnaire	NSFG Questionnaire	
		Female	Male
Ever had sex	Have you ever had sexual intercourse?	**Opposite Sex Partner** Vaginal Sex • At any time in your life, have you ever had sexual intercourse with a man, that is, made love, had sex, or gone all the way? *NOTE: Do not count oral sex, anal sex, heavy petting, or other forms of sexual activity that do not involve vaginal penetration. Do not count sex with a female partner.* • Has a male ever put his penis in your vagina (also known as vaginal intercourse)?	**Opposite Sex Partner** Vaginal Sex • Have you ever had sexual intercourse with a female (sometimes this is called making love, having sex, or going all the way)? • Have you ever put your penis in a female's vagina (also known as vaginal intercourse)?

continued

Question Category	YRBS Questionnaire	NSFG Questionnaire	
		Female	Male
Ever had sex (*continued*)	Have you ever had sexual intercourse? (*continued*)	Oral Sex • The next few questions are about oral sex. By oral sex, we mean stimulating the genitals with the mouth. Has a male ever performed oral sex on you? Have you ever performed oral sex on a male? That is, have you ever stimulated his penis with your mouth?	Oral Sex • The next few questions are about oral sex. By oral sex, we mean stimulating the genitals with the mouth. Has a female ever performed oral sex on you, that is, stimulated your penis with her mouth? • Have you ever performed oral sex on a female?
		Anal Sex • Has a male ever put his penis in your rectum or butt (also known as anal sex)?	Anal Sex • Have you ever put your penis in a female's anus or butt (also known as anal sex)?
		Same Sex Partner Oral Sex • Have you ever performed oral sex on another female? • Has another female ever performed oral sex on you?	**Same Sex Partner** Oral Sex • Have you ever performed oral sex on another male, that is, stimulated his penis with your mouth? • Has another male ever performed oral sex on you, that is, stimulated your penis with his mouth?
		Other Sex • Have you ever had any sexual experience of any kind with another female?	Anal Sex • Has another male ever put <u>his</u> penis in your anus or butt (receptive anal sex)? • Have you ever put <u>your</u> penis in another male's anus or butt (insertive anal sex)?

Question Category	YRBS Questionnaire	NSFG Questionnaire	
		Female	Male
Age at first sex	How old were you when you had sexual intercourse for the first time?	**Opposite Sex Partner** Vaginal Sex • That very first time that you had sexual intercourse with a male, how old were you? • The first time this occurred, how old were you? • Thinking back <u>after</u> your first menstrual period, how old were you when you had sexual intercourse for the first time? • How old were you when this first vaginal intercourse happened? **Same Sex Partner** Oral Sex • Thinking back to the <u>first time</u> you ever had oral sex or another kind of sexual experience with a <u>female</u> partner, how old were you?	**Opposite Sex Partner** Vaginal Sex • That very first time that you had sexual intercourse with a female, how old were you? • How old were you when this first intercourse happened? • The first time this occurred, how old were you? **Same Sex Partner** Any Sex • Thinking back to the <u>first time</u> you ever had any sexual experience with a <u>male</u> partner, how old were you?
Sequence of sexual acts		Opposite Sex Partner • Thinking back to when you had <u>oral</u> sex with a male for the first time, was it before, after, or on the same occasion as your first vaginal intercourse with a male?	Opposite Sex Partner • Thinking back to when you had <u>oral</u> sex with a female for the first time, was it before, after, or on the same occasion as your first vaginal intercourse with a female?

continued

Question Category	YRBS Questionnaire	NSFG Questionnaire	
		Female	Male
Lifetime sex partners	During your life, with how many people have you had sexual intercourse?	**Opposite Sex Partner** Any Sex • This next section is about your <u>male sex partners</u>. Now please think about any male with whom you have had vaginal intercourse, oral sex, or anal sex—any of these. • Thinking about your <u>entire life</u>, how many male sex partners have you had? Please count every partner even those you had sex with only once. **Same Sex Partner** • Thinking about your <u>entire life</u>, how many female sex partners have you had?	**Opposite Sex Partner** Any Sex • This next section is about your <u>female sex partners</u>. Now please think about any female with whom you have had vaginal intercourse, oral sex, or anal sex—any of these. • Thinking about your <u>entire life</u>, how many female sex partners have you had? Please count every partner even those you had sex with only once. Same Sex Partner • Thinking about your <u>entire life</u>, how many male sex partners have you had?
Recent sex partners[a]	During the past 3 months, with how many people have you had sexual intercourse?	**Opposite Sex Partner** Any Sex • Thinking about the <u>last 12 months</u>, how many male sexual partners have you had in the 12 months since [date]? Please count every partner, even those you had sex with only once in those 12 months. Vaginal Sex • Thinking of your male partners in the last 12 months, with how many of them did you have <u>vaginal intercourse</u>?	**Opposite Sex Partner** Any Sex • Thinking about the <u>last 12 months</u>, how many female sexual partners have you had in the 12 months since [date]? Please count every partner, even those you had sex with only once in those 12 months. Vaginal Sex • How many different females have you had sexual intercourse with in the past 12 months, that is, since [date]? • Thinking of your female partners in the last 12 months, with how many of them did you have <u>vaginal intercourse</u>?

Question Category	YRBS Questionnaire	NSFG Questionnaire	
		Female	Male
Recent sex partners[a] (*continued*)		Oral Sex • Thinking of your male partners in the last 12 months, with how many of them did you have oral sex? Anal Sex • Thinking of your male partners in the last 12 months, with how many of them did you have anal sex? **Same Sex Partner** Any Sex • Thinking about the last 12 months, how many female sexual partners have you had in the 12 months since [date]? Please count every partner, even those you had sex with only once in those 12 months.	Oral Sex • Thinking of your female partners in the last 12 months, with how many of them did you have oral sex, either giving or receiving? Anal Sex • Thinking of your female partners in the last 12 months, with how many of them did you have anal sex? **Same Sex Partner** Any Sex • Thinking about the last 12 months, how many male sexual partners have you had in the 12 months since [date]? Please count every partner, even those you had sex with only once in those 12 months. Oral Sex • Thinking of your male partners in the last 12 months, with how many of them did you have oral sex? Anal Sex • Thinking of your male partners in the last 12 months, with how many of them did you have receptive anal sex where he put his penis in your anus (butt)? • Thinking of your male partners in the last 12 months, with how many of them did you have insertive anal sex where you put your penis in his anus (butt)?

continued

Question Category	YRBS Questionnaire	NSFG Questionnaire	
		Female	Male
Substance use and sexual behavior	Did you drink alcohol or use drugs before you had sexual intercourse the last time?		
Condom use at last sex	The last time you had sexual intercourse, did you or your partner use a condom?	**Opposite Sex Partner** Any Sex • The very last time you had any type of sex—that is, vaginal intercourse or anal sex or oral sex—with a male partner, was a condom used? Vaginal Sex • Was a condom used the last time you had vaginal intercourse with a male? Oral Sex • Was a condom used the last time you performed oral sex on a male? Anal Sex • Was a condom used the last time you had anal sex with a male?	**Opposite Sex Partner** Any Sex • The very last time you had any type of sex—that is, vaginal intercourse or anal sex or oral sex—with a female partner, did you use a condom? Vaginal Sex • Did you use a condom the last time you had vaginal intercourse with a female? Oral Sex • Did you use a condom the last time a female performed oral sex on you? Anal Sex • Did you use a condom the last time you had anal sex with a female? **Same Sex Partner** Any Sex • The very last time you had any type of sex—that is vaginal intercourse or anal sex or oral sex—with a male or female partner, was a condom used? • Was that last sexual partner male or female?

Question Category	YRBS Questionnaire	NSFG Questionnaire Female	Male
Condom use at last sex (*continued*)			Oral Sex • Did you use a condom the <u>last time</u> you had oral sex with a male? Anal Sex • Did you use a condom the <u>last time</u> you had receptive anal sex with a male? • Did you use a condom the <u>last time</u> you had insertive anal sex with a male?
Pregnancy prevention at last sex[b]	The last time you had sexual intercourse, what one method did you or your partner use to prevent pregnancy? (Select only one response.)	**Opposite Sex Partner** Vaginal Sex • The last time you had intercourse with [partner] in [date], did you or he use any method? • Is the reason you did not use a method of birth control because you, yourself, wanted to become pregnant? • And your partner, did he want you to become pregnant? • Which method or methods did you or he use?	**Opposite Sex Partner** Vaginal Sex • That last time that you had sexual intercourse with your [wife/partner], did <u>you, yourself</u> use any methods to prevent pregnancy or sexually transmitted disease? • That last time, what methods did <u>you</u> use? • That last time that you had sexual intercourse with your (wife/partner), did <u>she</u> use any methods to prevent pregnancy or sexually transmitted disease? • That last time, what methods did <u>she</u> use?
Sex of sexual contacts[c]	During your life, with whom have you had sexual contact?	• Have you ever had any sexual experience of any kind with another female?	• Have you ever had any other sexual experience of any kind with another male?
Sexual orientation[c]	Which of the following best describes you?	• Which of the following best represents how you think of yourself?	• Which of the following best represents how you think of yourself?

[a]"Recent sex partners" refers to the last 3 months in the YRBS and last 12 months in the NSFG.

[b]The YRBS asks only about pregnancy prevention; the NSFG asks about both pregnancy and sexually transmitted infection (STI) prevention.

[c]Included in the YRBS since 2015.

SOURCE: Generated by the committee from YRBS questionnaires for 1991–2019 (CDC, 2018) and NSFG codebooks for 2015–2017 (CDC, 2019).

REFERENCES

Centers for Disease Control and Prevention (CDC). (2018). *YRBS Questionnaire Content—1991–2019*. Atlanta, GA: U.S. Department of Health and Human Services, Centers for Disease Control and Prevention, National Center for HIV/AIDS, Viral Hepatitis, STD, and TB Prevention, Division of Adolescent and School Health.

———. (2019). *2015–2017 NSFG: Public-Use Data Files, Codebooks, and Documentation*. Available: https://www.cdc.gov/nchs/nsfg/nsfg_2015_2017_puf.htm.

Appendix D

Public Information-Gathering Session Agenda

April 17, 2019 – 9:30am-5:00pm
National Academy of Sciences Building
2101 Constitution Avenue, NW Washington DC 20418

9:30-9:45   **Welcome and Introduction**
               Robert Graham, Committee Chair
               Nicole Kahn, Study Director

9:45-10:45   **Health Education Decision-Making in Public Education Systems**
               Moderator: Robert Graham, Committee Chair
               Panelists:
                    Robert Mahaffey, the Rural School and Community Trust
                    Wesley Thomas, District of Columbia Public Schools
                    Sandra Shephard, Prince George's County Board of Education

10:50-11:50   **Effective Measurement and Evaluation of Adolescent Behaviors/Behavior Interventions**
               Moderator: Robert Graham, Committee Chair
               Panelists:
                    Lisa Rue, cliexa
                    Ty Ridenour, RTI International
                    Elizabeth D'Amico, RAND Corporation

11:55-12:55   **Break: Lunch**

1:00-2:00   **Effective Elements of Programs Focused on Adolescent Behavior**
Moderator: Robert Graham, Committee Chair
Panelists:
      Aaron Hogue, the Center on Addiction
      Heather Hensman Kettrey, Clemson University
      Kim Robinson, Forum for Youth Investment

2:05-3:05   **Evaluating the Teen Pregnancy Prevention (TPP) Program and Sex Education Programs**
Moderator: Robert Graham, Committee Chair
Panelists:
      Randall Juras, Abt Associates
      Irene Ericksen, Institute for Research and Evaluation
      Jennifer Manlove, Child Trends

3:10-3:40   **Break**

3:40-4:40   **Discussion with Youth**
Moderator: Tammy Chang, Committee Member
Panelists:
      Richard Nukpeta, Mentor Foundation USA
      Shayna Shor, University of Maryland Health Center
         Peer Educator Program
      Natnael Abate, Promising Futures

4:45-5:00   **Closing**
Robert Graham, Committee Chair
Nicole Kahn, Study Director

Appendix E

Biosketches of
Committee Members and Staff

ROBERT GRAHAM (*Chair*) has spent his career in health policy and the management of health care organizations. He joined the U.S. Public Health Service in 1970, serving a total of 18 years during three tours of duty over the next 30 years. During this time, he was deputy director of the Agency for Healthcare Research and Quality (AHRQ) and the first administrator of the Health Resources and Services Administration (HRSA), holding the ranks of rear admiral and assistant surgeon general. He has long been associated with the medical specialty of family medicine, serving as CEO of the American Academy of Family Physicians from 1985 to 2000 and as an endowed professor of family medicine at the University of Cincinnati from 2005 to 2013. Throughout his career, Dr. Graham has written and spoken extensively about a number of critical topics in health policy, such as health care reform and the need for universal coverage, health workforce policy, and the organizational characteristics of effective health care systems. He received his undergraduate degree from Earlham College in 1965 and his medical degree from the University of Kansas in 1970.

RICHARD ADRIEN was an associate program officer on the Board on Children, Youth, and Families (BCYF) at the National Academies, providing research support for the Committee on Applying Lessons of Optimal Adolescent Health to Improve Behavioral Outcomes for Youth through August 2019. Prior to joining the National Academies, he provided technical assistance and research support on issues pertaining to equity, education, and youth development. Additionally, he has counseled youth in educational and community settings to help them identify and attain their career and educational goals. He received his Ed.M. in international education development from Columbia University and his M.Ed. in counseling from the University of Toronto.

PAMELLA ATAYI is a program coordinator on BCYF, providing logistical and administrative support for the Committee on Applying Lessons of Optimal Adolescent Health to Improve Behavioral Outcomes for Youth. She coordinates and oversees the work of support staff handling clerical, administrative, and logistical aspects of meetings. Ms. Atayi provides work direction and assists with the daily supervision of support staff. She also compiles and summarizes information for the development and revision of a variety of documents and participates in research efforts. She serves as liaison between programs and boards of the National Academies, and related external customers, members, and sponsors on clerical and administrative matters. Ms. Atayi was awarded the Sandra H. Matthews Cecil Award by the Institute of Medicine (now the Health and Medicine Division) in 2013, and the Espirit de Corps Award by the Division on Behavioral and Social Sciences and Education in 2017. She received her B.A. in English from the University of Maryland University College and a diploma in computer information systems from Strayer University.

ANGELA BRYAN is a professor of psychology and neuroscience at the University of Colorado Boulder. She is co-director of the CUChange Research Laboratory, where her research has focused on a transdisciplinary approach to the study of health and risk behavior and the development of interventions to improve health behaviors. Dr. Bryan capitalizes on the integration of basic scientific discoveries regarding biological predispositions associated with health and risk behavior (e.g., genetics and neurocognition) and applied intervention work to change behavior. Much of her work has focused on the reduction of substance use–related HIV/sexually transmitted disease (STD) risk behavior among adolescents. This work has been funded by several institutes of the National Institutes of Health (NIH), including the National Institute on Alcohol Abuse and Alcoholism (NIAAA), the National Institute on Drug Abuse (NIDA), and the National Institute of Nursing Research (NINR). She has more than 170 peer-reviewed publications and has been teaching health psychology, social psychology, research methods, and statistical methods to undergraduates and graduate students for more than 20 years. Dr. Bryan received her Ph.D. in social psychology with a quantitative emphasis from Arizona State University.

TAMMY CHANG is an assistant professor in the Department of Family Medicine at the University of Michigan and a practicing family physician. She is a health services researcher with a focus on adolescent health, specifically, breaking the cycle of poverty and poor health among adolescent mothers and their children. Her NIH-sponsored research is focused on improving access to reproductive health care and promoting healthy pregnancy weight gain among at-risk adolescents using text messaging, social media mining, and natural language processing (NLP). She is also the founding director of MyVoice, a national text-message poll of youth ages 14 to 24 that uses mixed methods and NLP with the goal of informing local and national policies in real time. She has published in several academic journals and received numerous awards, including the James C. Puffer, M.D./American Board of Family Medicine Fellowship at the National Academy of Medicine. Dr. Chang received her M.D. from the University of Michigan.

ROSALIE CORONA is a professor of psychology, director of clinical training, and founding director of the Latina/o Mental Health Clinic at Virginia Commonwealth University (VCU). Prior to joining the faculty at VCU, she worked as a research scientist at the University of California, Los Angeles (UCLA)/RAND Center for Adolescent Health Promotion. Her community-engaged research focuses on Latina/o and African American adolescents' health promotion and risk reduction, applying specific expertise in adolescent sexual health and substance use prevention. A theme throughout her scholarship is the role of family and culture in promoting adolescents' health behaviors. Dr. Corona's community-engaged research has progressed from an initial focus on identifying local health disparities and the associated risk and protective factors to the development, implementation, and evaluation of family-based prevention programs to address these disparities. She has been a principal investigator or co-investigator on projects funded by the Centers for Disease Control and Prevention (CDC), the National Heart, Lung, and Blood Institute (NHLBI), the National Cancer Institute (NCI), the National Institute of Child Health and Human Development (NICHD), and the Virginia Foundation for Healthy Youth. Her reputation as a community-engaged research scholar and teacher has resulted in multiple editorial board invitations, and her accomplishments have also been recognized locally and nationally. Dr. Corona received her Ph.D. in clinical psychology from UCLA.

TAMERA COYNE-BEASLEY is a professor of pediatrics and internal medicine, director of the Division of Adolescent Medicine, and vice chair of Pediatrics for Community Engagement at the University of Alabama Birmingham. She has expertise and training in adolescent medicine, medical management, epidemiology, and public health. She also completed a preventive medicine residency/fellowship with the U.S. Department of Health and Human Services in the Office of Disease Prevention and Health

Promotion and a Robert Wood Johnson Clinical Scholars program with a focus on health services research. Dr. Coyne-Beasley is a past president of the Society for Adolescent Health and Medicine, an international multidisciplinary organization dedicated to promoting the optimal health and well-being of adolescents and young adults. Her academic efforts, community work, policy development, and research have focused on adolescent health, resiliency and risk behaviors, mental health and suicide prevention, health promotion and disease prevention, injury prevention, reducing health disparities, increasing immunizations, improving health care access, community-based participatory and engaged research, practice-based research, sexual and reproductive health, and pregnancy prevention. Dr. Coyne-Beasley received her M.D. from Duke University.

BONNIE HALPERN-FELSHER is a professor in the Division of Adolescent Medicine in the Department of Pediatrics at Stanford University. As a developmental psychologist with training in adolescent and young adult health, she has focused her research on social, environmental, cognitive, and psychosocial factors involved in health-related decision making, perceptions of risk and vulnerability, health communication, and risk behavior. Funded by NIH and many foundations, her research has emphasized understanding and reducing adolescent tobacco use, alcohol and marijuana use, and risky sexual behavior. She is a core member of the University of California, San Francisco (UCSF) Center for Tobacco Control Research and Education, a project coleader for the NIH and Food and Drug Administration (FDA)–funded UCSF Tobacco Center of Regulatory Science, and a co–principal investigator for the new UC Merced Cannabis and Nicotine Policy Center. Dr. Halpern-Felsher's research and committee work have been instrumental in setting policy at the local, state, and national levels. She has served as a consultant to a number of community-based adolescent health promotion programs and has been an active member of several national campaigns to understand and reduce adolescent risk behavior. She has also served on five National Academies committees and contributed to three surgeon general reports, all focused on reducing adolescent risk behavior and promoting health. Dr. Halpern-Felsher received her Ph.D. in developmental psychology from the University of California, Riverside.

JEFFREY W. HUTCHINSON is a retired U.S. Army colonel currently working in Austin, Texas, as CEO of The Wade Alliance, LLC, a leadership, diversity, and inclusion consulting organization, and a BCYF member at the National Academies. As an adolescent medicine specialist and previous associate dean and chief diversity officer at the Uniformed Services University of the Health Sciences, he has a unique perspective on adolescent behavior and health equity. His career includes combat in Iraq, clinical leadership, and executive membership on the American Academy of Pediatrics council on communication and media. With 25 years of experience caring for children, teens, young adults, and service members, he applies the intersection of systems with humanism and communication to help teens and parents. He is an advocate for addressing the social determinants of health disparities and has published in several academic journals. Dr. Hutchinson received his M.D. from the University of California, San Francisco.

REBEKAH HUTTON is a program officer in BCYF, providing research support for the Committee on Applying Lessons of Optimal Adolescent Health to Improve Behavioral Outcomes for Youth since August 2019. Previously, she was an education management and information technology consultant working on projects in the United States as well as Haiti, Equatorial Guinea, and Djibouti. She has also worked as a program manager and researcher at the National Center on Performance Incentives at Vanderbilt University, studying whether teacher pay for performance has a measurable impact on student outcomes, and as an English language lecturer in Tourcoing, France. During her time with BCYF, she has worked on projects focused on fostering the educational success of children and youth learning English; reducing child poverty; and promoting the mental, emotional, and behavioral health of children and youth. She received her M.Ed. degree from Vanderbilt University in international education policy and management and a B.A. degree from the University of Tennessee in French language and literature.

NICOLE F. KAHN is a program officer in BCYF and study director for the Committee on Applying Lessons of Optimal Adolescent Health to Improve Behavioral Outcomes for Youth. Before joining the National Academies, Dr. Kahn worked as a social research specialist with the Carolina Population Center at the University of North Carolina at Chapel Hill, where she collaborated on research projects focused on postsecondary educational attainment, adolescent sexuality, and childhood and adolescent precursors of adult chronic disease. She has also worked as a project researcher at the Georgetown University Center for Child and Human Development in Washington, DC, and served as a Head Start teacher with the Teach for America program in Phoenix, Arizona. She received her M.Ed. in early childhood education from Arizona State University and her Ph.D. in maternal and child health from the Gillings School of Global Public Health at the University of North Carolina at Chapel Hill, where she studied the sexual experiences and related health outcomes of marginalized populations from adolescence to adulthood.

VELMA MCBRIDE MURRY is a professor in the Departments of Health Policy and Human and Organizational Behavior in the School of Medicine and Peabody College and endowed Lois Autrey Betts chair of education and human development at Vanderbilt University, as well as a former BCYF member. Dr. McBride Murry is a nationally recognized expert in examining ways in which racism affects the processes, behaviors, and health outcomes of families, and has conducted developmental, prospective studies on African American parents and youth for more than 15 years to identify proximal, malleable protective factors that deter youth risk engagement. This work has advanced current knowledge of the impact of contextual factors, particularly racism, on African American family functioning through the development of novel strength-based family prevention interventions, including the Strong African American Families and Pathways for African American Success programs. Both programs are designed to enhance parenting and family processes to in turn encourage youth to delay age at sexual onset and the initiation and escalation of alcohol and drug use. Dr. McBride Murry has published more than 125 papers and received more than 25 external grants to fund her research activities. She received her Ph.D. in human development and family studies from the University of Missouri, Columbia.

SANDRA JO WILSON is a principal associate in the Social and Economic Policy Division at Abt Associates. Dr. Wilson's work focuses on approaches to developing and packaging actionable evidence on effective programs. She is an expert in the design and conduct of meta-analyses and systematic reviews and has broad content knowledge relevant to youth prevention programs. She currently leads a project supported by the Assistant Secretary for Planning and Evaluation to develop practice guidelines for youth programs using a common components approach to evidence-based practice. In addition, she is project director for the Prevention Services Clearinghouse, an evidence clearinghouse established by the Administration for Children and Families to systematically review research on programs and services intended to provide enhanced support to children and families and prevent foster care placements. Dr. Wilson's functional skills include research design, research synthesis, statistical analysis, product development, and technical assistance. Her domain expertise includes school-based violence prevention, juvenile delinquency, high school dropout prevention, college/career readiness, and early childhood education. Dr. Wilson received her Ph.D. in policy development and program evaluation from Vanderbilt University.